R0006375772

D1444074

RIT - WALLACE LIBRARY
CIRCULATING LIBRARY BOOKS

OVERDUE FINES AND FEES FOR <u>ALL</u> BORROWERS

*Recalled = $1/ day overdue (no grace period)
*Billed = $10.00/ item when returned 4 or more weeks overdue
*Lost Items = replacement cost+$10 fee
*All materials must be returned or renewed by the duedate.

Compression
for Clinicians

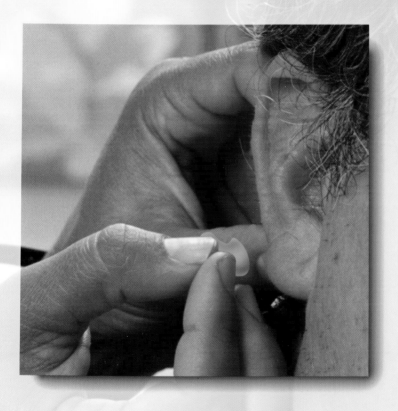

Theodore H. Venema

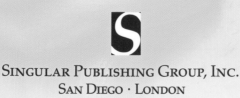

SINGULAR PUBLISHING GROUP, INC.
SAN DIEGO · LONDON

Compression for Clinicians

A Singular Audiology Text
Jeffrey L. Danhauer, Ph.D.
Audiology Editor

COMPRESSION
FOR
CLINICIANS

Ted Venema, Ph.D.

Unitron Industries Ltd.
Kitchener, Ontario, Canada

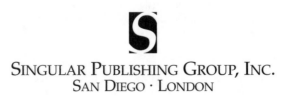

SINGULAR PUBLISHING GROUP, INC.
SAN DIEGO · LONDON

Singular Publishing Group, Inc.
401 West A Street, Suite 325
San Diego, California 92101-7904

Singular Publishing Ltd.
19 Compton Terrace
London N1 2UN, UK

Singular Publishing Group, Inc., publishes textbooks, clinical manuals, clinical reference books, journals, videos, and multimedia materials on speech-language pathology, audiology, otorhinolaryngology, special education, early childhood, aging, occupational therapy, physical therapy, rehabilitation, counseling, mental health, and voice. For your convenience, our entire catalog can be accessed on our website at **http//www.singpub.com**. Our mission to provide you with materials to meet the daily challenges of the everchanging health care/educational environment will remain on course if we are in touch with you. In that spirit, we welcome your feedback on our products. Please telephone **(1- 800-521-8545)**, fax **(1-800-774-8398)**, or e-mail **(singpub@mail.cerfnet.com)** your comments and requests to us.

© 1998 by Singular Publishing Group, Inc.

Typeset in 10/12 Century by So Cal Graphics
Printed in the United States of America by Bang Printing
Second Revised Printing March 1999

All rights, including that of translation, reserved. No part of this publication may be reproduced, stored in a retrieval system or transmitted in any form or by any means, electronic, mechanical, recording, or otherwise, without the prior written permission of the publisher.

Library of Congress Cataloging-in-Publication Data

Venema, Ted.
    Compression for clinicians/by Ted Venema.
        p.   cm. — (A Singular audiology textbook)
    Includes bibilographical references and index.
    ISBN 1-56593-973-5 (pbk.   :   alk. paper)
    1. Hearing aid—Fitting.   2. Compression
(Audiology)   3. Hearing aids—Design and construction.
I. Title.   II. Series: Singular audiology text.
    [DNLM: 1. Hearing Aids.   2. Prosthesis Fitting-
-methods.   3. Cochlea—physiology.   4. Loudness
Perception.   5. Equipment Design.   WV 274 V456c 1998]
RF300.V46 1998
617.8'9—dc21
DNLM/DLC
for Library of Congress   98-28845
                                                                                              CIP

Contents

Preface

The purpose of this book is to connect, hook, or tie together concepts about compression and hearing aids that we as clinicians have all heard before. My intent is not to present the new, cutting-edge research in hearing aids nor to focus on the "hot" topic of digital-signal-processing (DSP) hearing aids. I hope, instead, to clearly explain and make understandable the many buzz words of the 1990s relating to compression and hearing aids for those who fit hearing aids for a living. I think that, if this objective is met, one can apply these concepts of compression to the fitting of any hearing aid, regardless of its technical origins.

Much has changed in our knowledge of the cochlea and hearing aids since the late 1980s. The discovery of otoacoustic emissions (OAEs) heralded a new way of describing the role of the outer hair cells as distinct from that of the inner hair cells. This more detailed description of the otherwise inaccessible cochlea in turn affected the way compression was designed for those with sensorineural hearing loss.

Before 1990, when I left clinical audiology to pursue a doctorate in audiology, I was accustomed to fitting linear hearing aids using fitting methods based on the half-gain rule. While busy at school, things arrived in the world of hearing aid technology, that is, the K Amp™ circuits, programmable hearing aids, multichannel hearing aids, and completely-in-canal hearing aids. Several new "suprathreshold" hearing aid fitting methods also began to be introduced in most of the more popular periodicals. When I re-entered the real world, I certainly had a lot of catching up to do. This book is a product of my learning process. It is an attempt to clarify and organize the many commonplace concepts that have formed the landscape of our clinical field.

The book is aimed squarely at the area that unites audiologists, hearing aid dispensers, and students: namely, the clinical field of fitting hearing aids. This book is intended to be direct and easy to read, with readily accessible information. If the goal of this book is reached, clinicians and students should not have to scour the index only to find the core ideas buried within a thickly worded text.

The book has six chapters and three appendixs. Chapter 1 provides a short description of the fascinating cochlea and highlights its hair cell functions as a "two-way street." These relatively recent additions to our cochlear knowledge base are the underlying basis of some types of compression, as discussed in later chapters. Chapter 2 describes a big-picture view of the field of hearing aid fitting and offers a contrast to optometry and the fitting of lenses for the eye. The vast differences between these two fields help explain why we have so many hearing aid fitting methods in the first place. Chapter 3 offers a description of loudness growth and the necessity of compression and also provides a short description of three popular suprathreshold fitting methods. These newer fitting methods are based on loudness growth and assume compression in hearing aids. The heart of the book is Chapter 4, which outlines, compares, and contrasts the many types of compression available to clinicians today. In this chapter, the clinical applications of the various types of compression are also described. Chapter 5 provides a short discussion on the terms "programmable" and "digital" in hearing aids, and describes two current digital hearing aids that use compression. Chapter 6 concludes with some thoughts about what hearing aids can and cannot do. The gross function of a compression hearing aid is contrasted to the exquisite function of the active, living cochlea. Types of compression are condensed and categorized for mild-to-moderate and for severe-to-profound hearing losses, and an example of a multichannel WDRC hearing aid is described. Questions are raised about the implications of fitting with one method as opposed to another. Despite our recent advances in hearing aid circuitry and fitting sophistication, we still have a long way to go. Appendix A is a short description of the various amplifier classes used in today's hearing aids. Appendixes B and C include two previously published articles that may be of clinical interest to readers.

Acknowledgments

I want the people at Unitron Industries, Ltd. to know that I am grateful for the help and opportunities they gave me over the past few years since I began working there in the summer of 1995. In particular, I want Paul Darkes, formerly of Unitron and now at Phonak, to know that I really appreciate all that he taught me about hearing aids. I could never have written Chapter 4 without his input. Paul was my mentor and friend while we worked together for 2 years at Unitron. Paul always showed remarkable patience with my immensely slow speed of learning. He also continues to laugh at my really dumb jokes.

My wife, Laura Venema, took on a lot of work with our family and put up with my many absences so that I could write this book. Thank you, Laura, my love; I couldn't have done it without you.

Dedication

This book is dedicated to my daughter, Kathryn Ashley, who was born March 26, 1994 in Opelika, Alabama. Kathryn is our special child. Her mother, Laura Kathryn, her younger sister, Angela Dawn, and I believe she is really an angel who is here to remind us that things are not always as they seem.

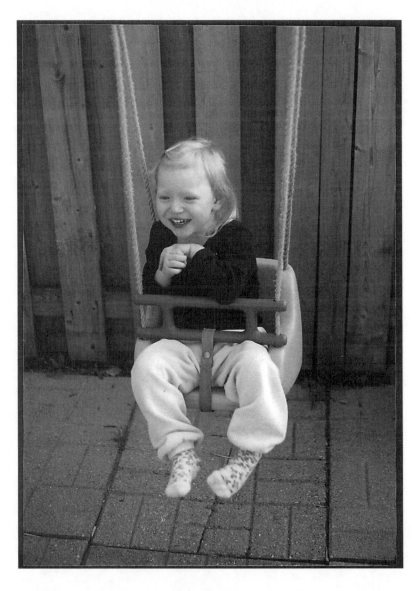

CHAPTER 1

The Cochlea, Hair Cells, and Compression

This chapter covers some relatively recent concepts about the cochlea and its function, which have everything to do with compression. This material is fundamental to a comprehensive understanding of compression in hearing aids.

The cochlea is described in general, broad strokes, with particular attention to the roles of the inner versus the outer hair cells. Each of these sets of hair cells do completely different things. We now know that the outer hair cells help the inner hair cells sense soft sounds and that the outer hair cells are usually damaged during normal wear and tear before the inner hair cells deteriorate. These different roles have ramifications for the types of compression that can be used in fitting people with hearing aids. The typical end result of outer hair cell damage is a sensorineural hearing loss of around 50 dB HL; this degree of hearing loss is consistent with the most common hearing loss today, which is presbycusis. The fitting of hearing aids for presbycusis may need to imitate the role of the outer hair cells in particular. This chapter outlines the problems posed by hair cell damage; later chapters discuss the goals of amplification for various degrees of hearing loss and the means of applying compression to different clinical populations.

The cochlea (from the Greek *Kochlias* for snail shell) is one of the most complicated organs in the body, but its purpose can be explained in one sentence: It changes sound into electricity and electricity is the language the brain understands. The relative size of the cochlea in diagrams is often drawn far too large and is depicted as being about the size of an eyeball. This is fundamentally false; the cochlea is really quite small, about the size of the tip of your little finger. It has only 2½ turns in humans; in other mammals, the cochlea may look different. In the chinchilla, for example, the cochlea has 3½ turns.

As a complex organ, the cochlea and its functions are very difficult to understand. It might be easier to understand the relationships between its labyrinths, or chambers, and how they function if the cochlea could be unrolled into a straight line (Figure 1–1). Essentially, it consists of a tube within a tube. Each tube is filled with fluids that have very different chemical compositions. The smaller of these tubes is soft-walled, long and narrow, and is closed at one end. This tube is situated lengthwise within a larger, wider fluid-filled, hard-walled cave. The word "cave" is used here because the larger, outside chamber is completely housed within bone.

There is one thing to note about the relationships between the smaller tube within the larger cave: The tube completely separates the cave into an upper and a lower chamber. It is as if the wider cave is bent in the middle and folded in half. The small, soft-walled tube is located in the center of the larger cave, thus separating the larger cave into upper and lower portions. This relationship results in three chambers: a lower hard-walled cave with a soft ceiling (scala tympani), a middle soft-walled chamber (scala media), and a higher hard-walled chamber with a soft floor (scala vestibuli). The upper and lower portions of the cave are connected only at the bend. This bend is the apex or small tip of the cochlea; the fluid in the wide tube can move around the bend through a passage called the helicotrema.

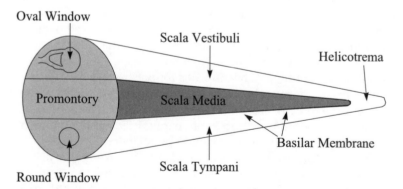

Figure 1–1. An unrolled cochlea shows the scala vestibuli and scala tympani wrapped around the scala media. These two chambers are continuous and are joined by the helicotrema. Thus, they both share the same fluid, which is very different in composition than that inside the scala media.

In reality, the cochlea is coiled, or rolled up, and therefore occupies a very small length in the skull. In keeping with the analogy of the cochlea as a cave, it might be a good idea to think of it as a coiled hole or labyrinth, augered into bone. One might as well look at a hole in the ground and then ask for the hole itself to be dug out, so it can be seen standing like a cup. It is no wonder, then, that the human cochlea is very difficult to extract and show as a single unit.

The coils of the cochlea, as mentioned earlier, are filled with two very different kinds of fluid. A cross-section of one coil of the rolled up cochlea reveals the three chambers described. The smallest chamber with the soft walls looks like a small triangle situated in the middle. The top and bottom chambers correspond to the hard-walled cave that is bent in half (Figure 1–2).

The top chamber, the scala vestibuli, can be said to "begin" at the oval window and "end" at the helicotrema. Similarly, the scala tympani begins at the round window of the cochlea and ends at the helicotrema. The hair cells of the cochlea are located in the middle cham-

Cross Section of the Human Cochlea

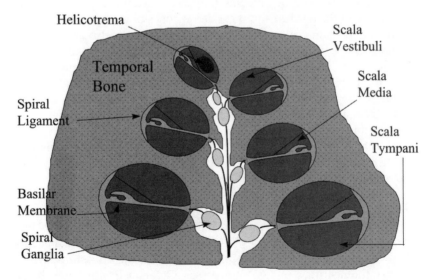

Figure 1–2. The human cochlea is often shown as if it exists as a snail-shaped presence, ready for easy excision and examination. Unlike the cochlea of many small mammals, however, the human cochlea is a labyrinth of coils completely embedded in bone (gray area in the figure). Therefore, the human cochlea is especially inaccessible.

ber, the scala media. The "floor" upon which the hair cells are situated in the cochlea is called the basilar membrane. It divides the bottom chamber, the scala tympani, from the middle chamber, or scala media. The basilar membrane runs along the whole length of the cochlea, from the base to the apex (see Figure 1–1). When "unrolled," the basilar membrane is about 24–35 mm long (Yost, 1994).

Incoming sound, conducted by the middle ear bones that terminate at the oval window of the cochlea, moves the body of fluid that fills the scala vestibuli and scala tympani. The fluid motion is in the form of a *traveling wave*, with a peak of maximal indentation at one location or another along the length of the cochlea. The outer walls of the scala vestibuli and scala tympani are bone, whereas the walls of the scala media are membranous. As a result, the only thing that can give or be displaced by the traveling wave peak is the scala media. The scala media is thus *indirectly* stimulated by incoming sound from the fluid movement within the scala vestibuli and scala tympani. Hair cells are activated when incoming sound stimulates or bends the middle chamber at some particular place or point. When hair cells are stimulated at the base, or wide end, of the cochlea, we hear high-frequency sounds; when hair cells are stimulated at the apex, or narrow peak, of the cochlea, we hear low-frequency sounds.

As mentioned earlier, the tiny human cochlea is completely embedded in one of the hardest and most dense bones of the body, the petrous portion of the temporal bone (Figure 1–2). The word "petrous" originates from the Greek language, and has the same meaning as the name "Peter," which means "hard, like a rock." The cochlea is, therefore, quite inaccessible for physical examination, at least while a person is alive. The cochleas of chinchillas have commonly been studied because, in these rodents they stick out into the middle ear space like a small honeycomb; these cochleas are much easier to excise and examine than those of humans. Only the relatively recent discovery of otoacoustic emissions (OAEs) (Kemp, 1978) has provided us with a glimpse or a window into the real-time physiology, or function, of the human cochlea.

Otoacoustic emissions have shown us that the function of the outer hair cells (OHCs) is very distinct from that of the inner hair cells (IHCs). The OHCs are very mechanical; they actually stretch and shrink (Brownell, 1996). They are very busy little cells and because they work so hard, emit a by-product: otoacoustic emissions, which are like the hearing process "in reverse." Otoacoustic emissions begin at the OHCs and go out from the cochlea, back through the ossicular chain to tympanic membrane (TM). The TM acts as a loudspeaker, converting the mechanical movement of the middle ear ossicles back into sound waves. It is bizarre but true that the ear can make sound as well as receive it!

Knowledge about the different IHC and OHC functions directly relates to compression in hearing aids. As is shown in later chapters, some types of compression are designed specifically to imitate the function of the OHCs. In this way, one can strive to amplify sounds to sound as natural as possible for persons with hearing loss.

INNER AND OUTER HAIR CELLS: STRUCTURE AND FUNCTION

The IHCs are rounded or flask-like in shape like small pears. Their "hairs," or stereocilia, do not touch the tectorial membrane (see Figure 1–3). The IHCs communicate mostly with VIII nerve (CN VIII) fibers

A Simple View of the Organ of Corti

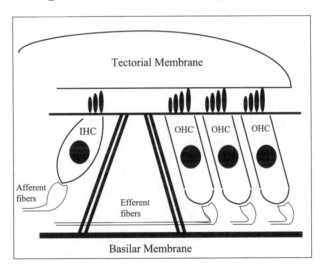

Figure 1–3. The inner (IHCs) and outer hair cells (OHCs) of the cochlea are very different in shape, and they also serve very different functions. The stereocilia of the IHCs, unlike those of the OHCs, do not touch the tectorial membrane. The figure shows afferent fibers only at the IHCs and efferent fibers only at the OHCs, because, for the most part, these are the roles of the respective hair cells. In reality, however, a closer inspection reveals that the arrangement is not so simple. Some efferent fibers also are attached to the afferent fibers that terminate on the IHCs. Some afferent fibers are also attached to the OHCs, themselves.

and terminate at the lower brainstem. More specifically, the CN VIII fibers exit the right and left cochleas and terminate at the right and left cochlear nuclei, which are located on the lower brainstem, where the medulla meets the pons.

Simple intuition suggests that, if things look different, they probably do different things. As Figure 1–3 shows, the IHCs and OHCs look different from each other and they do, indeed, have very different roles. The IHCs are mostly "afferent," which means that they send sound information *to* the brain (Brownell, 1996). Without IHCs, information about sound cannot be sent on to the brain and there is, essentially, no hearing. With damage to the IHCs, "brain-going" information is affected and a person may have difficulty understanding speech in quiet and especially with background noise (Killion, 1997c).

The OHCs are completely different. Unlike the IHCs, the OHCs are cylindrical, or shaped like test tubes. Their "hairs," or stereocilia, are embedded in the bottom of the tectorial membrane (Figure 1–3). They communicate mostly through a bundle of neuron fibers, which leave the lower brainstem and terminate at the OHCs. These fibers are called the "olivocochlear bundle." The fibers of the olivocochlear bundle begin at the right and left superior olivary complexes in the lower brainstem, run along side of the afferent CN VIII fibers, and end at the OHCs in both the opposite (crossed or contralateral) and same-side (uncrossed or ipsilateral) cochleas (Brownell, 1996).

The OHCs are "efferent," which means they take information *from* the brain back to the cochlea. They receive messages from the superior olivary nuclei in the lower brainstem (and probably higher centers as well), which tell them to either elongate or shrink and this mechanical action changes the mechanical properties of the basilar membrane at specific spots. For soft incoming sounds, the OHCs play an especially strong role, as they mechanically enable the IHCs to sense soft sounds and "sharpen" the peak of the traveling wave (Brownell, 1996). Without the OHCs, we would have a moderate degree (40 to 60 dB HL) of sensorineural hearing loss (Berlin, 1994). It follows that if someone has a severe hearing loss (e.g., 80 dB HL), then there is probably both IHC and OHC damage.

At this time no one really knows exactly how the whole afferent IHC and efferent OHC feedback loop, or system, works (Bobbin, 1996; Killion, 1996b, Norris, 1996). For example, which afferent messages get *to* the superior olivary complexes in the lower brainstem that, in turn, are sent back in an efferent direction to the OHCs? We do know the basics, however. The OHCs amplify soft incoming sounds and "sharpen" or fine tune the traveling wave of the cochlea. More on this is discussed later.

Basilar Membrane and Passive Traveling Wave

The name of a Hungarian Nobel peace prize winner, Georg von Békésy, has become synonymous with the concept of a traveling wave peak that stimulates hair cells in specific areas along the basilar membrane. This cochlear membrane forms the boundary between the scala media and the scala tympani of the cochlea and is the "floor" upon which the hair cells are located. The basilar membrane ranges from about 24 to 35 mm in length (Yost, 1994). It is interesting to note that the basilar membrane is wider (.42 to .65 mm) at the narrow apex of the cochlea and is narrower (.8 to .16 mm) at the wider base of the cochlea (Figure 1–4). The small apex of the cochlea thus has more room, or "real estate," to accommodate about five outer hair cell rows than at the large base of the cochlea, where there are about three rows. This also is why there are *more* than three times as many OHCs as IHCs.

At the apex of the cochlea, the wide basilar membrane has more mass and is more flaccid than it is at the base of the cochlea. The narrow basilar membrane at the base of the cochlea has less mass and is stiffer. High frequencies move best through stiff objects that have less mass;

Cochlear Physiology: Traveling Wave

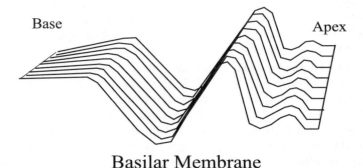

Base   Apex

Basilar Membrane

Figure 1–4. The basilar membrane is mostly narrow (and stiff) at the relatively wide base of the cochlea; it is widest and with more mass (and is less stiff) at the small apex of the cochlea. These physical properties determine which hair cells are stimulated by incoming low-frequency or high-frequency sounds. The wider shape at the apex of the cochlea allows for more than three rows of outer hair cells, which are often shown on diagrams.

low frequencies move best through objects that have more mass and less stiffness. This is why high frequencies produce a traveling wave that stimulates the base and low frequencies produce a traveling wave that stimulates the apex of the cochlea.

Von Békésy (1960) described the traveling wave as having a rounded peak, but more recent studies have shown that this dull, rounded peak is found in cochleas that have damaged hair cells (Brownell, 1996). A traveling wave with a dull, rounded peak presents problems when trying to figure out how the cochlea fine "tunes" for frequencies that are close together. For example, if humans can hear frequencies from 20 to 20,000 Hz, then how can a dull, rounded traveling wave allow us to distinguish the difference between, say, 500 Hz and 520 Hz? Some thought might lead one to question the gross nature of hair cell stimulation with such a rounded peak. How does the cochlea do precise fine tuning? According to Brownell (1996), a colleague of von Békésy's (Gold, 1948), proposed that the OHCs had an active role in sharpening the traveling wave peak, but this explanation was dismissed from lack of evidence. The CN VIII was known to have sharp tuning curves, and von Békésy believed that a fine frequency resolution thus took place further "up" the auditory system chain of command.

OHCs and Active Traveling Wave

The concept of the active versus the passive cochlea is relatively new; only within the past 10 years has this view of the cochlea become a real part of the clinician's knowledge base. Through the discovery of otoacoustic emissions, we now know that the OHCs do indeed have an *active* role in cochlear mechanics.

An active (as opposed to passive) traveling wave with OHC involvement is shown in Figure 1–5. In this example, the low-frequency hair cells are receiving most of the traveling wave excitation. The peak of the traveling wave is the site of greatest hair cell stimulation, but without the OHCs, the peak is rounded. Given a hearing range of from about 20 to 20,000 Hz, such a dull, rounded traveling wave peak stimulates many different frequencies at once.

The IHCs are stimulated when the traveling wave bends the basilar membrane and this occurs with incoming sounds of 40 to 60 dB SPL (Bobbin, 1996; Killion, 1996b). Softer sounds, like 10 dB SPL, somehow stimulate the OHCs to "do their mechanical thing," which is to help the IHCs sense the soft sounds. Without the OHCs, the IHCs can sense sounds from about 40 to 60 dB SPL up to the level of physical sensation or total loudness discomfort; by themselves, the IHCs cannot sense sounds below these levels. Damage to the OHCs thus implies a hearing

Outer Hair Cell Contributions to the Traveling Wave

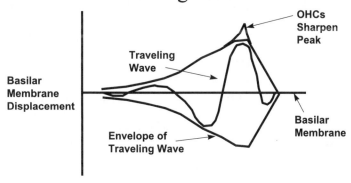

Figure 1–5. The outer hair cells amplify and sharpen the peak of the traveling wave. With a pointed peak, the traveling wave looks like an inverted CN VIII tuning curve. The basilar membrane is the "floor" upon which the inner and outer hair cells are situated. On the left, are the high-frequency hair cells at the base of the cochlea; on the right are the low-frequency hair cells at the apex of the cochlea. The traveling wave bends the basilar membrane, which in turn excites the hair cells. Note that the envelope of the traveling wave is asymmetrical.

loss of 40 to 60 dB, and this is often the degree of hearing loss found with presbycusis.

As mentioned earlier, in addition to amplifying soft incoming sounds for the IHCs, the mechanical action of the OHCs also "sharpens" the peak of the traveling wave (Brownell, 1996). With their mechanical movements, the OHCs actually change the physical properties of the basilar membrane around the passive peak of the traveling wave, so that its peak is sharpened. A passive traveling wave with a dull, rounded peak may not enable one to distinguish among frequencies that are close together. Is it any wonder then, that the person with OHC damage may have poorer speech discrimination ability?

The whole active cochlear mechanism is extremely complex. Think of the speed at which the OHCs have to move to influence the reception of sounds by the IHCs; the OHCs would have to be able to move or react very quickly. In fact, the OHCs do have the ability to move faster than any muscle can (Brownell, 1996). Killion (1996b) suggested that with soft incoming sounds, the OHCs shrink. Because their stereocilia are actually embedded in the tectorial membrane, the OHCs pull the membrane down when they shrink, and this shortens the gap between the tectorial membrane and the tips of the IHC stereocilia. When the tips of the IHC stereocilia can touch the tectorial membrane, they can be bent or sheared and thereby send sound information to the brain. So for soft sound inputs, the OHCs mechanically help the IHC stereocilia to make contact so they can be sheared or bent by the tectorial membrane.

The *active* traveling wave in Figure 1–5 has a shape that is a mirror image of the tuning curves of CN VIII fibers. In this figure, it appears that the OHCs literally "pick up" and "sharpen" the peak of the traveling wave.

In summary, the OHCs have a twofold purpose: they amplify soft incoming sounds below 40 to 60 dB SPL, allowing the IHCs to sense them, and they also fine tune the frequency resolution of the cochlea. With damage to the OHCs, we have a corresponding loss of their function. As mentioned earlier, this results in a 40 to 60 dB (mild-to-moderate) sensorineural hearing loss. If the hearing loss is greater than mild-to-moderate in degree, then there is probably both IHC and OHC damage.

The Traveling Wave and Upward Spread of Masking

Note that the traveling wave in Figure 1–5 is asymmetrical, with a long, shallow "tail" and a relatively "steep" wave front. If low-frequency hair cells are stimulated with a relatively large amplitude traveling wave, then the entire basilar membrane moves and many hair cells from higher frequency regions are also stimulated. On the other hand, if high-frequency hair cells are stimulated with a large amplitude traveling wave, the low-frequency hair cells are not so easily stimulated.

The asymmetry of the traveling wave has important implications for audiometry. For example, when testing someone with a "reverse" hearing loss (moderate hearing loss for the low frequencies and normal hearing for the high frequencies), the actual low-frequency hearing loss *could* be worse than indicated on the audiogram (Thornton & Abbas, 1980). Low-frequency, pure-tone testing at levels greater than 50 dB HL may inadvertently stimulate the normally functioning high-frequency hair cells, causing the subject to respond.

The asymmetry of the traveling wave is a cochlear explanation for what is commonly known as the "upward spread of masking." Classic masking experiments have also shown the relatively greater efficiency of low-frequency versus high-frequency maskers (Bess & Humes, 1995). In short, low frequencies mask high frequencies better than high frequencies mask low frequencies. The upward spread of masking also seems to wreak havoc for the person with hearing aids when listening in background noise. Perhaps this is why hearing aid fitting methods often tend to prescribe relatively less amplification for the low frequencies than for the high frequencies.

DAMAGED HAIR CELLS AND HEARING LOSS

To contrast normal and damaged hair cells, look at the electron micro-scope photographs in Figures 1–6 and 1–7. Healthy normal IHCs and OHCs are seen in Figure 1–6. According to Yost (1994), there are about 3,500 IHCs in each cochlea. On top of each IHC are about 40 to 60 "hairs," or stereocilia, which are arranged in shallow "Vs." Each cochlea has about 12,000 OHCs. On top of each OHC are about 100 to 150 stereocilia, which are arranged like "horseshoes" in three or more rows.

Figure 1–7 shows damaged hair cells. Note that the damage is most-ly confined to the OHCs. Loss of the OHCs causes loss of their function, which results in a more passive, dull and less active, sharp traveling wave. In audiometry, this translates into a mild-to-moderate sensorineur-al hearing loss. Because the OHCs are very mechanical (i.e., they move a lot), they use lots of oxygen. These highly mobile hair cells are very sensitive to the insults that life throws at them over the years of one's ex-istence. Most hair cell damage thus begins with the OHCs and later on is evident in the IHCs (Willott, 1991). If a sensorineural hearing loss is about 50 dB HL or less, it can usually be assumed that the damage is con-

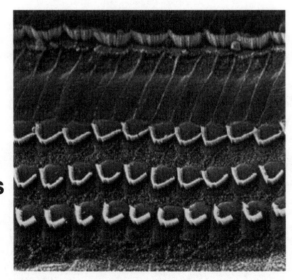

Normal
Inner
&
Outer
Hair Cells

Figure 1–6. An electron microscope photograph of normal, healthy human inner and outer hair cells. (From *The Biology of Hearing and Deafness* (p. 21), by R. Harrison, 1988, Springfield IL: Charles C. Thomas, Publisher. Copyright 1988 by Charles C. Thomas, Publisher. Reprinted with permission.)

Impaired Outer Hair Cells

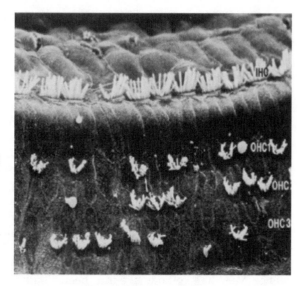

Figure 1–7. An electron microscope photograph of damaged hair cells. Most of the damage is confined to the outer hair cells. From *The Ear: Some Notes on Structure and Function*, by H. Engstrom and B. Engstrom, 1988, p. 12, Vaerloese, Denmark: Widex. Copyright by Widex. Reprinted with permission.

fined to the outer hair cells. If the hearing loss is, for example, 80 dB HL, then it is safe to assume that the damage involves both IHCs and OHCs.

Presbycusis: The Most Common Type of Hearing Loss

The word "presbycusis" is composed of two Greek words: "presby," which means "elders," and "cusis," which means "hearing." Presbycusis is reminiscent of the word "presbyterian," which means "church of the elders," and "presbyopia," which means "vision of the elders."

Presbycusis, or hearing loss found in aging ears, manifests itself as a mild-to-moderate sensorineural hearing loss, and it is by far the most common type of hearing loss in our society today. About 80% of the people living in the United States with hearing loss have presbycusis (Hull, 1995). As the baby-boom generation ages, the demographics show that there is a large "bubble," or segment, of people who are increasing in age and so the average age of our population is also increasing. Therefore, we should expect to see an increase of clients having presbycusis in the future.

Most presbycusis results in a mild-to-moderate sensorineural hearing loss, which is consistent with OHC damage. People with presbycusis often have a hearing loss that is mild in degree for the low frequencies and moderate in degree for the high frequencies.

Jerger, Chmiel, Stach, and Spretnjak (1993) compared hearing loss configurations in men and women between the ages of 50 and 89 years. They found that, in general, men often have a more steeply sloping hearing loss than women, with a greater degree of hearing loss in the high frequencies and less hearing loss in the low frequencies. For women, the greater hearing loss in the low frequencies might result from degeneration of the stria vascularis, which affects blood supply to the cochlear hair cells. For men, the greater hearing loss in the high frequencies might show the interaction of work-related noise-induced hearing loss (NIHL) and presbycusis.

NIHL also causes damage to the OHCs (Engstrom & Engstrom, 1988), especially when the noise to which the person is exposed is constant. However, according to Borg, Canlon, and Engstrom (1995) and Killion (1997c), sudden, sharp noises like loud gunshots will cause both IHC and OHC damage. As mentioned earlier, OHC damage may result in some trouble understanding speech in background noise; but the IHCs send most sound information to the brain. If these IHCs are damaged, then the message to the brain may in and of itself be "garbled," resulting in greater difficulty separating speech from background noise, even when clients are properly aided (see also Chapter 2)! Noise in our society is gradually becoming more of an issue for concern, especially as general awareness of NIHL filters through to the general public.

Hearing Aids for the Damaged Cochlea

Figure 1–8 illustrates the normal versus damaged hair cells seen in Figures 1–6 and 1–7, respectively. Hearing aids must meet a daunting goal in trying to imitate the action of the normal cochlea. Unfortunately, this cannot be done. At present trying to restore normal hearing with hearing aids is like trying to pick up needles with mittens on. The amplified sound must get through the middle ear to the cochlea and stimulate damaged or remaining hair cells. We are not simply sending amplified sound to intact hair cells. If we were, hearing aid fittings would be more like fitting eyeglasses.

Hearing aids cannot grow new hair cells. Although a few experiments have shown that we can reproduce hair cells in birds (Ryals, 1995), as we go higher up in the animal kingdom, hair cells are more difficult to reproduce. When we can grow new hair cells, hearing aids will become

Hearing Aids Do Not Grow New Hair Cells

A
hearing
aid
cannot
fill
in
the
spaces

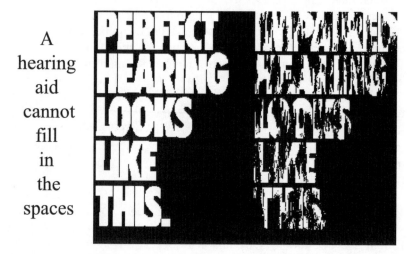

Figure 1–8. A verbal illustration of the normal and damaged hair cells shown in Figures 1–6 and 1–7. With normal hearing, there are many hair cells. With hearing loss, hair cells are damaged and/or there are fewer cells. Can amplification of fewer hair cells possibly imitate the action of many haircells? At most hearing aids will make the white areas of the figure (right side) become whiter and the black areas become darker, but they cannot fill in the spaces. (Adapted from a poster. Copyright held by The Canadian Hearing Society, Toronto, Ontario, Canada. Adapted with permission.)

extinct and the reader (and author) will be looking for other work. However, because that will not likely happen in the near future, emphasis needs to be placed on developing the best hearing aids possible.

The results of a sharpened traveling wave can be intuitively surmised: It is probable that frequency discrimination and hearing in noise are improved (or normal) with a sharpened peak. No hearing aid presently available can sharpen the peak of the traveling wave like the OHCs do. But the OHCs are also known to increase cochlear sensitivity by at least 40 dB (Killion, 1996b). For those with OHC damage, perhaps hearing aids should focus amplification on sounds below 40–50 dB. The cochlea is a nonlinear organ. The softer the input, the more it amplifies. Perhaps this is a rationale for using nonlinear amplification. Recent knowledge about the function of the cochlea has everything to do with compression in hearing aids.

SUMMARY

■ The OHCs sharpen the peak of the traveling wave and amplify soft incoming sounds below approximately 40 to 50 dB SPL. With hearing aids today, we can imitate only the second of these functions.

■ The OHCs are mechanical in nature, they use a lot of oxygen, and they are usually the first to die or be damaged. Loss of the OHCs results in a mild-to-moderate degree of hearing loss. If hearing loss is severe, there is probably damage to the IHCs as well as the OHCs.

■ The most common type of hearing loss today is presbycusis, which is typically mild to moderate in degree. For the population with presbycusis, we need to try to imitate OHC function, and to do so we must amplify soft sounds by a lot and intense sounds by little or nothing at all.

RECOMMENDED READING

Ear & Hearing, 11(2), 1990. The whole issue is devoted to OAEs.

Killion, M. C. (1995). Talking hair cells: What they have to say about hearing aids. In C. I. Berlin (Ed.). *Hair cells and hearing aids* (pp. 125–172). San Diego: Singular Publishing Group.

Ryals, B. M. (1995). Hair cell regeneration: Is it just for the birds? *The Hearing Journal, 48*(7), 10–83.

C H A P T E R   2

Why So Many Different Hearing Aid Fitting Methods?

Hearing aid fitting methods are used to determine how much amplification to provide for clients having specific hearing losses. But for any specific hearing loss, there are many hearing aid fitting methods that can be used, and each one will lead to a prescription of somewhat different amounts of amplification at different frequencies. The student of hearing aids is often puzzled as to why so many different methods are used to fit hearing aids. The seasoned practitioner/dispenser of hearing aids also wonders about the same thing. Each year, the newest fitting methods and their rationales are presented at conferences. The newest fitting methods are usually based on restoring normal loudness growth to the impaired ear (see Chapter 3), and they consistently address *compression* in hearing aids. The older threshold-based fitting methods are largely based on *linear* hearing aid circuitry.

Linear hearing aids are called "linear" because they provide the same gain for all input sound levels. On an input-output graph, the line showing the function of linear hearing aids is straight or linear (until the maximum power output is limited and peak clipping occurs). Compression hearing aids, on the other hand, provide *different* amounts of gain for different input sound levels. There are many different types of compression hearing aids and for any one of these, the line on an input-output graph showing the function of a compression hearing aid is not straight. Hence, compression hearing aids are often called nonlinear hearing aids. More is discussed about input-output graphs and also the wide topic of compression in Chapter 4.

As the years pass, in all health-related fields there is a constant exposure to new technology. But, in the hearing health care discipline we are also exposed to constantly evolving fitting methods. One thing is certain: Regarding hearing aids, the fitting method(s) one learns at school will not necessarily represent all of the methods practiced at any future time in the real world by most clinicians. Thus, clinicians are often overwhelmed by the necessity of the constant learning process.

LENSES FOR THE EYE VERSUS HEARING AIDS FOR THE EAR

Fitting hearing aids is very different from fitting eyeglasses or contact lenses. More specifically, fitting hearing aids for presbycusis is a very different thing from fitting lenses for presbyopia. Some answers as to why we use so many different hearing aid fitting methods can be found if we look to another health science: optometry. Sometimes defining who we are not helps us to get a better idea of who we are.

The general public is well aware that eyeglasses work better for the eye than hearing aids do for the ear. For the optometrist and the client, the fitting of lenses is either done correctly or incorrectly. The repercussions of an improper fitting of lenses are usually headaches or blurred vision. If this is not rectified, the person simply cannot wear the lenses. People do not normally go to visual rehabilitation classes, nor do they routinely return to optometrists for further instruction to learn how to use their eyeglasses after the initial fitting. After the lenses are prescribed, the person simply chooses the color and style of glasses he or she wants and the story usually ends there.

The general public is also aware that most typical vision problems result from an improper focus of light on the retina, which is situated against the back of the eyeball. In the simplest terms, the retina does for the eye what the organ of Corti does for the ear. The retina changes light into electricity, because electricity is the language the brain understands. A refocusing of light on an intact retina with properly fitted lenses is similar to fitting a person with conductive hearing loss with hearing aids. For the client with poor vision, incoming light that does not focus correctly on the retina has to be properly conducted, or refocused so it can get *to* where it should go. For the client with conductive hearing loss, sound simply has to be amplified or conducted so that it can get through the middle ear, *to* where it has to go (i.e., the hair cells of the inner ear).

If optometrists had the same job as audiologists or hearing aid dispensers, they would most often be seeing clients with scratched or damaged retinas (Figure 2–1). In these cases, even the proper focus of light on the retina will not bring about "normal" vision. This is the situation for the clinician fitting hearing aids. Only for conductive hearing loss is the cochlea intact. For the most part, hearing aids are fit on people with sensorineural hearing loss, with the hair cells of the cochlea damaged. This makes the problem more difficult than simply amplifying sound for a conductive hearing loss.

The hair cells of the cochlea are the "retina" of the ear (see Figure 2–1). Because most hearing loss results from damage to this "retina" of hearing, the fitting of hearing aids is different from the fitting of lenses, and the benefits of hearing aids are not quite so obvious, especially to those who wear them! If the benefits of hearing aids are not clear to the client or if the hearing aids are physically uncomfortable, then clients simply will not wear them.

Hearing aids make incoming sounds louder, so persons with hearing loss can hear them. Persons with mild hearing losses are fit with low-gain hearing aids, and those with severe hearing losses are fit with high-gain hearing aids; persons with high-frequency hearing losses are

Fitting the Eye versus Fitting the Ear

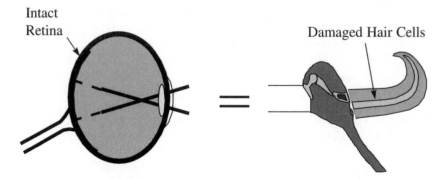

Intact
Retina

Damaged Hair Cells

The "Retina" of the Ear is the Organ of Corti

Figure 2–1. Optometrists refocus light toward an intact end-organ, the retina. Audiologists must fit a damaged end-organ of hearing, the cochlea. The "retina" of the ear is the organ of Corti.

generally fit with high-frequency emphasis hearing aids, and those with low-frequency hearing losses are generally fit with low-frequency emphasis hearing aids. But beyond these obvious facts, what are the implications for clients if hearing aids are prescribed with one fitting method versus another? Will they get headaches? Will they truly hear "better" when fit with one fitting method versus another? It is truly interesting that no one hearing aid fitting method has been proven to be the "best" for any condition, let alone speech intelligibility in noise. Here we reach the great impasse of hearing aid fitting methods: Choosing a fitting method is really a matter of *choice*, not really a matter of correct versus incorrect.

What Are We Actually Doing When Fitting Hearing Aids?

When immersed in the clinical fitting of hearing aids, clinicians can sometimes get bogged down by the absorption of new information. Think about what we are doing when we fit hearing aids. First, consider that, unlike the eyeball which is situated on the front of the face, the cochlea is buried almost an inch "behind" the outer ear or pinna. With the output sound from the hearing aids, we are smashing the eardrum with increased pressure and driving the middle ear ossicles harder than they were ever really meant to be driven, in the hope that the increased sound pressure will somehow increase the amplitude of the traveling wave and excite remaining undamaged hair cells in the cochlea.

As mentioned in Chapter 1, outer hair cell (OHC) damage will cause the "active" sharpened traveling wave to become "passive" and more rounded. The result of this "dulled" traveling wave is a mild-to-moderate sensorineural hearing loss. The traveling wave cannot be sharpened with hearing aids at this time. We can, however, make small steps to "imitate" the function of the OHCs with hearing aids by deliberately increasing cochlear sensitivity to soft sounds below 40 to 50 dB SPL. "Normal" cochlear function is certainly not restored with hearing aids; if it was, hearing aid fittings would be far more successful and fitting methods would be far fewer.

Hearing Speech Better Is What Most People Want From Hearing Aids

Among modern day humans, hearing is mostly a communicative sense we use to receive speech. Therefore, in the big picture of hearing and hearing aids, speech figures front and center. Vision, however, is mostly an environmental sense we use to negotiate and find our way in the physical world. Here it must be said that for the deaf community, vision and language share a special relationship because vision is the primary mode of receiving sign language. Deaf people use their eyes in more capacities than most hearing people could imagine. Witness the experience necessary to test persons with severe and profound hearing loss; they might raise a hand to a pure-tone presentation just because they see the examiner's shoulder move when the audiometer interrupter button is pushed.

For most people with hearing loss who wear hearing aids, hearing is the primary sense they employ to receive speech. For these people, the importance of *speech understanding in noise* cannot be overestimated. For students of hearing loss and hearing aids, this problem may not be self-evident or easy to comprehend. After all, those with typical hearing have problems hearing speech when there is a lot of background noise, but we get over it by yelling louder. Why is this then such a problem for those who wear hearing aids? If hearing aids amplify the speech and the background noise together, then why are people with hearing aids not in the same position as those with normal hearing?

To better understand why those with hearing aids often complain bitterly about understanding speech in noise, two things are important to acknowledge: the unique acoustic properties of the sound called speech and the results of hair cell damage.

Improving speech understanding in noise is not as simple a matter as making a steady—state pure tone audible amid environmental background noise or the hubbub of surrounding speech. The ongoing pops and fizzes of frontal, consonantal sounds, the combinations of tonal elements, and the temporary closures of our vocal tracts defy an easy characterization and an easy separation from background noise, even with the assistance of mathematical algorithms used in current digital signal processing (DSP) hearing aids (see Chapter 5). Speech consists of complicated acoustic signals that are rapidly changing in intensity and frequency over time.

Speech is meant to be understood, but all of its flowing, changing elements must first be audible. To be audible, aided speech has to be discerned as separate from aided background noise. Given the combination of (1) the nature of cochlear hair cell damage and (2) the present hearing aid technology, this goal is not readily achieved.

As described in Chapter 1, damage to the OHCs results in a mild-to-moderate hearing loss of around 50 dBHL; the damage also results in a broadened traveling wave, without the active sharpening that is normally provided by the OHCs. This may in turn result in poorer frequency discrimination and resolution for the client (Willott, 1991). However, provided that the hearing aids do not distort too much, a person with OHC damage may still do fairly well when listening to speech in background noise (Killion, 1997c). Again, as discussed in Chapter 1, damage to the OHCs often precedes damage to the IHCs.

Damage to the IHCs, however, has an even more dramatic effect on the ability to understand speech in background noise, because this results in a loss of afferent sound information to the brain from the cochlea. Persons with IHC damage lose the ability to separate or extract the speech from the background noise, and they need an abnormally large ratio of speech intensity relative to noise intensity (improved signal-to-noise ratio) to understand speech in noise (Killion, 1997c). According to Killion (1997b, 1997c) and Killion, Schulein, Christensen, Fabry, Revit, Niquette, & Chung (1998), to understand 50% of speech, speech has to be at least as or more intense (perhaps as much as 2.5 dB) as background noise. Those with cochlear hair cell damage, especially IHC damage, require an *additional* 5 or 6 dB of speech in relation to background noise to understand 50% of the speech. In general, each 1 dB of speech relative to the background noise level results in about a 10% improvement in speech intelligibility. This implies that persons with IHC damage cannot be expected to do well when listening to speech in background noise, even when aided with the best available technology. The best thing hearing aids can do in this case is to not cause any further problems (Killion, 1997c).

In general then, listening to speech in the presence of background noise is a real problem for those with sensorineural hearing loss, especially for those with IHC damage. Even the best or most promising of our current technology, such as digital signal processing (DSP) hearing aids, cannot effectively subtract or *remove* background noise from the desired speech. When DSP algorithms try to actually subtract background noise from speech, they also take out tiny, valuable pieces of sounds, or speech cues that are necessary for accurately perceiving speech. Hearing aids cannot replace the incredible function of normal hearing; when they try to separate speech from background noise completely, they tend to "throw the baby out with the bath water."

In a rather humorous experiment (Bentler & Duve, 1997), an 1880s speaking tube was tested against two recent popular digital hearing aids on the Auditec Speech in Noise™ test at a cocktail party. The background noise levels were a moderate 83 dB SPL. The results were about equal for all three "contestants." This finding suggests that we have not yet solved the problem of removing background noise from speech, even with DSP.

It is no wonder that hearing aid fitting methods have not been as exact a science as optometric fitting methods. Aside from an inability to sharpen the traveling wave, the target of amplification is speech, which is often spoken when there is also surrounding background noise. Unfortunately, hearing aids today are not especially adept at separating speech from background noise. Without hearing aids, people with hair cell damage hear soft, garbled speech that is difficult for them to separate from the background noise; with our present-day hearing aids they hear louder garbled speech. Audibility of speech may be improved, but *clarity* of speech is not necessarily improved with hearing aids, especially in the presence of background noise.

A Word About Directional Microphones

One way to increase the signal-to-noise ratio for those with hearing loss is with directional microphones. These types of microphones provide a way to work *around* the problem of damaged cochlear hair cells. It is presently impossible to work *through* the problem, that is, to repair the damaged cochlea or to subtract noise from target speech by DSP technology. To give a geographical analogy, directional microphones can be considered a way of avoiding the necessity of boating over the treacherous Niagara Falls; they provide a parallel canal, in this case, the Welland Canal, to sail around the obstacle.

Directional microphones have been in existance for about 50 years and have been used in BTEs and ITEs for about 20 years (Preves, 1997). Directional microphones in hearing aids are intended to enhance the signal-to-noise ratio by picking up a greater amount of sound from the front of the listener, as compared to sounds that arrive from other angles. However, these directional microphones have not enjoyed much acceptance, mainly because they have not provided clients with the hoped-for benefits. Killion et al. (1998) mention that in BTEs the directional microphone typically has not provided as much benefit as the "low-tech" solution of cupping one's hand behind the ear to hear better in difficult listening situations. Furthermore, the typical hearing aid directional microphone cannot be switched off and on at will, and this has been a serious oversight on the part of manufacturers (Preves, 1997). A notable exception to these problems is the Audiozoom™ by Phonak, which has overcome these obstacles (Kuk, 1996). Another exception is the D-MIC™ for the ITE, by Etymotic Research (Killion et al., 1998).

The benefit of a directional microphone for speech intelligibility can be demonstrated through the use of a combination of measures: the articulation index based directivity index (AI-DI). The AI-DI results in a single number in decibels by which to measure the overall effectiveness of a directional microphone (Roberts & Schulein, 1997; Killion, et al. 1998). It shows in decibels, the signal-to-noise ratio improvement for listening to speech that would result if the background noise were turned down by that amount (ER-44 D-MIC data sheet, 1997).

The directivity index (DI) is the difference between the microphone's sensitivity to sounds directly in front of the listener compared to sounds that may come from any other direction. Figure 2–2 shows four polar plots, which illustrate the directionality of the typical onmidirectional microphone versus the directionality of three directional microphones. The polar plots are idealized, that is, they do not include the real effects of head shadow, sound diffraction, and so on (if they did, they would be more ragged and bumpy in shape). The omnidirectional microphone picks up sound equally in all directions. In Figure 2–2 it has a round polar plot and a DI of zero. Three different types of directional pat-

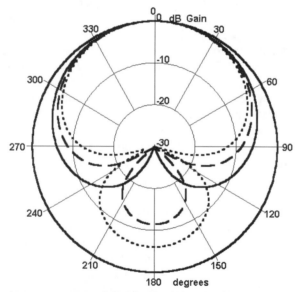

Polar Plots for Directional Microphones

Figure 2–2. Idealized polar plots are shown for the omnidirectional (the widest, outside circle) and also for various types of directional microphones. The polar plot that looks like a heart is from a "cardioid" directional microphone. The polar plot with the smallest rear lobe is from the supercardioid directional microphone, and the remaining polar plot is from the hypercardioid directional microphone. According to Preves (1997), the cardioid microphone has a DI of 4.8 dB, the supercardioid directional microphone has a DI of 5.7 dB, and the hypercardioid directional microphone has a DI of 6.0 db.

terns are illustrated by the other three polar plots. All of these are equally sensitive to sounds originating from in front of the listener, but they have unequal sensitivity to sounds coming from the other directions.

The polar plots shown in Figure 2–2 do not show frequency, and it is important to acknowledge that the DI varies for different frequencies. The clues or cues for recognizing speech are found more at some frequencies than at others, and, therefore, a different weighting should be given for some frequencies than for others. Accordingly, the DI is weighted according to frequency by the articulation index (AI). Figure 2–3 shows an audiogram with 100 dots, which represent the acoustic energy of speech. Each dot represents 1% of the speech cues required for optimal speech recognition (Mueller & Killion, 1990). It is not sur-

Articulation Index

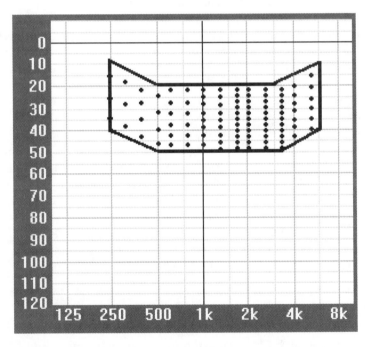

Figure 2–3. The count-the-dot audiogram, where each dot represents 1% of the cues necessary to recognize speech. The dots below one's hearing thresholds represent the speech that would be audible to the person; the dots above one's hearing thresholds represent the speech that is not audible. The count-the-dot audiogram can be used as a way to assign weight or importance to frequency regions of speech. Note. From An Easy Method For Calculating the Articulation Index, by Mueller, H.G., & Killion, M.C. (Figure 1, p. 15) *The Hearing Journal, 43*(9). Copyright 1990 by Williams & Wilkins Publishing Company. Reprinted by permission.

prising that the frequencies between 1000 and 4000 Hz have the most dots, and are, therefore, given the most weight. The DI-AI results from the weighting of the AI, applied to the DI at each frequency.

The AI-DI for a particular directional microphone is typically between 0 to 6 dB. This may seem small, but recall that a single decibel increase in signal-to-noise ratio results in close to 10% in speech intelligibility (Killion (1997b, 1997c) and Killion, et al. 1998). An AI-DI of 3 dB would, according to this calculation, result in a 30% increase in speech intelligibility!

EVOLUTION OF HEARING AID FITTING METHODS

As discussed earlier, OHC damage, the most common type of cochlear hair cell damage, results in a mild-to-moderate degree of sensorineural hearing loss. What has not been specifically addressed is the issue of loudness tolerance for intense sounds, which is often true for those with sensorineural hearing loss. More will be discussed on this topic in Chapter 3. At this point, it is sufficient to note that for most people with sensorineural hearing loss, the "ceiling" of loudness tolerance for intense sounds does not change significantly; it is the "floor," or the ability to hear soft sounds, that changes most. The loss of hearing sensitivity thus changes at only one end of the hearing range or spectrum; thus, sensorineural hearing loss does *not* result in a need to have all sounds amplified by the *same* amount.

The first hearing aid fitting methods arose out of a compromise between (1) the knowledge that for sensorineural hearing loss, sensitivity for soft sounds is reduced, although the loudness perception for intense sounds is not, and (2) the available hearing technology at the time, which amplified soft and intense sounds by the same amount.

A Short History of Hearing Aid Technology

In the first half of the 20th century, hearing aids had a remarkably limited frequency response and, therefore, were fit mostly on persons with flat conductive hearing losses or gently sloping sensorineural hearing losses. Most were "body" style hearing aids that had a flat frequency response that dropped off above 2000 Hz. Individuals with flat hearing losses could be fit with these hearing aids, but clients with steeply sloping high-frequency sensorineural hearing loss, often called "tractor deafness," were told nothing could aid this type of hearing loss. Choosing a hearing aid for a particular client was a simple matter of deciding whether he or she needed one.

Around 1900, hearing aids were carbon based, which means the microphone was filled with carbon granules (Hodgson, 1986). Incoming sound pressure made patterns in the resistance of the carbon granules, which resulted in patterns of electrical current that were then transduced back into sound by a magnetic "earphone," or receiver. The microphone and receiver had to have overlapping resonances and so the carbon hearing aids had a narrow frequency response with a single peak.

The 1920s saw the development of vacuum tube hearing aids that were much more powerful than carbon-based hearing aids, but also quite large and inflexible in frequency response. The earlier ones had crystal microphones, which were much more efficient than the carbon microphones. Vacuum tube hearing aids required *two* batteries: one to heat the filaments inside the vacuum tubes and another to provide the general power for amplification. Due to their large size, these vacuum tube hearing aids could not be worn on the ear.

In the 1950s the transistor replaced the vacuum tube and hearing aids became much smaller with better high-frequency emphasis (Hodgson, 1986). Because transistors were so much smaller than vacuum tubes, they required far less power and, thus, the battery size became smaller. Frequency responses also became more flexible and could provide anything from a broad- or wide-frequency response to more high-frequency emphasis. Over the past two decades, the typically sharp peaks in the frequency responses and the distortion seen in earlier hearing aids have been reduced. Interestingly, even though hearing aid distortion has been reduced, as late as the 1970s it was sometimes still so bad that, even people with *normal* hearing had problems when they wore hearing aids and listened to speech in background noise (Killion, 1997c).

Body-style hearing aids gave way to behind-the-ear (BTE) hearing aid styles in the late 1950s, and these soon became the norm. The BTE style also became incorporated in a hearing aid–eyeglass combination. This may have had some cosmetic appeal, but the hearing problem remained when wearers took off their glasses, they also removed their hearing aids. In the 1960s, in-the-ear (ITE) styles began to appear. The first ITEs were modular, which meant that they snapped onto a custom-made earmold. Later developments led to nonmodular ITEs, with circuits built into earmold shells. Cosmetic desires by consumers for hearing aids that were least visible drove the manufacturing industry to emphasize the production of ITEs. In the early 1980s, smaller canal hearing aids began to appear, and in the 1990s, the even smaller completely-in-canal styles have become ever more popular.

Another major development in hearing aids have been the types of circuits that have become available; namely, the nonlinear or, "compression," hearing aid circuits. Prior to the 1970s, linear circuits prevailed (and some persist to this day), but beginning in the early 1970s nonlinear, or compression, hearing aid circuits began to replace or augment manufacturer offerings of linear hearing aid circuitry. At first, compression was offered as a solution for those with hearing loss who also experienced discomfort at low loudness levels. Much more is discussed about compression in later chapters. For now, the concept of "linear" needs to be elaborated, because it is the *interaction* between linear circuitry in hearing aids and the exquisitely nonlinear cochlea that gave rise to the vast array of fitting methods that we have today.

Hearing Aid Fitting Methods Based on Linear Technology

The first hearing aid fitting methods were based on or assumed the use of linear circuitry in hearing aids. To understand linear hearing aids, it is important to be familiar with the most basic formula for hearing aids: Input + Gain = Output (see Figure 2–4). "Input" is whatever sound enters a hearing aid, "gain" is the amount of amplification given to the input by the hearing aid, and "output" is the sum total of sound that travels from the hearing aid and into one's ear.

An output intensity of 120 dB sound pressure level (SPL) is usually uncomfortably loud for both those with normal hearing and individuals with sensorineural hearing loss. Normal conversational speech averages at about 70 dB SPL. If a hearing aid supplies 45 dB of gain to that 70 dB, then its output approaches 120 dB SPL. For a person with a similar uncomfortable listening level, this may be the maximum gain we can add to the intensity of average, ongoing speech before the discomfort level is reached. As long as the input sounds are about 70 dB or less, the output sounds from the hearing aid will remain below the uncomfortable listening level for that person. If the input level rises above 70 dB, then the added gain of 45 dB will result in an output that exceeds 120 dB SPL, and the person will have discomfort.

A hearing aid circuit that provides the same amount of gain for any and all input intensity levels is known as "linear" (Figure 2-4). That is, the aid produces 1 dB of output for each decibel of input (a 1:1 ratio) up to a certain maximum output limit. For example, if a hearing aid has 50 dB of linear gain at full-on volume, then it will provide 50 dB of gain to 10 dB SPL input sounds as well as to 70 dB SPL inputs. The corresponding outputs will be 60 dB SPL and 120 dB SPL, respectively. The first output would be tolerable for most individuals, but the

Linear Amplification

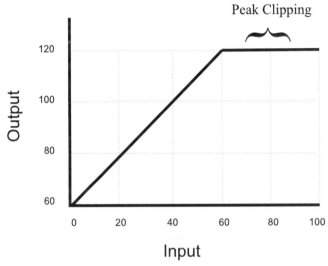

Figure 2–4. With linear hearing aids, the output increases entirely along with the input. In this example, the gain of the linear hearing aid is 60 dB. For 20 dB inputs, the output is 80 dB; for 60 dB inputs, the output is 120 db; for 100 dB inputs, the output would be 160 dB (if not for output limiting)! People with sensorineural hearing loss usually cannot stand much more than about 120 dB SPL, and so linear circuits introduce "peak clipping." This means that any output more than 120 dB SPL gets clipped, or "cut off."

second probably would not. When hearing aid outputs exceed a wearer's uncomfortable listening level, the remedy of linear circuitry is to "clip the peaks" of the maximum output. This is usually accomplished with a maximum power output (MPO) control, or peak clipper, on the hearing aid.

The main problem with limiting the output with peak clipping is that when the output sound exceeds the set MPO, the hearing aid becomes saturated and distorts the sound and the *quality* of listening is sacrificed. If a hearing aid provides 60 dB of gain and the MPO is set to around 120 dB SPL, then the typical speech inputs of 70 dB SPL will constantly drive the hearing aid into saturation; and this will result in poor sound quality. Linear hearing aids were the "state of the art" in hearing aid technology until the mid-1970s and even in the 1980s, most hearing aid fittings involved linear circuitry.

A Short History of Fitting Methods

Hearing aid fitting methods have evolved over the past half century as a result of a mixture of hearing aid technology available at any particular time and the experimental trials and errors of scientific inquiry. Carhart (1946) developed a clinical comparative approach of trying several hearing aids on the same person to determine the "best" one for speech recognition and which one the person "liked" the best. His approach involved various speech test measures in unaided and aided conditions with each of several different hearing aids. Typically at that time, clinicians relied on their own internal criteria, which were often based on personal experience with particular hearing aid models. It soon became clear that it was difficult to teach this method to someone else and to generalize the criteria from one clinic to another. Clinicians began to feel the need for a systematic *prescription* approach to fitting hearing aids, a system that could be followed by anyone anywhere.

Can't We Just "Mirror" the Audiogram With Gain?

"Mirroring" the audiogram simply means providing as much gain as the hearing loss, itself. If a person's hearing loss is 20 dB HL for the low frequencies and 50 dB HL for the high frequencies, a mirror of this hearing loss would then imply providing 20 dB of gain for the lows and 50 dB of gain for the highs. Although many clinicians tried, it became clear that we cannot simply "mirror" the audiogram with full gain, at least not with linear hearing aid amplification. Figure 2–5 (left panel) shows an audiogram with a pronounced high-frequency hearing loss. The right panel of Figure 2–5 shows the same audiogram flipped upside-down, so the concept of mirroring the audiogram might become more clear. If it were possible simply to amplify sound by the degree of the hearing loss, then there would be only one fitting method needed, and one would fit hearing aids "correctly" or "incorrectly," and new fitting methods would not surface every year. To students learning about hearing aids and to practicing clinicians this would be a relief.

"Mirroring" the audiogram seems intuitively correct, because we could make all thresholds "0" for the person's hearing loss. That is, zero dB HL input sounds would then become "just barely audible," much like they are for persons with "perfect" hearing. Slightly more intense sounds, like 10 dB HL, would become audible at a sensation level of 10 dB, and so on. But what about more intense sound inputs, like speech? Can we amplify all sounds equally? Not with linear hearing aids.

"Mirroring" the audiogram with full linear gain could only be closer to the truth, if the tolerance for loudness grew along with the

"Mirror" the Audiogram with Full Gain?

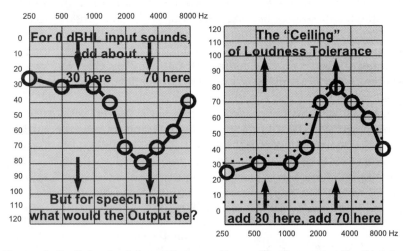

Figure 2–5. "Mirroring" the audiogram with amplifications seems like the intuitive thing to do. But if this were true, there would only be one fitting method! The left panel shows the typical audiogram as obtained in most clinics. The right panel shows intensity now read as "up," similar to the way we read hearing aid specification sheets. The dotted lines show 5 dB HL sounds that could be amplified so they are audible to the person. But could speech be amplified by the same amount?

hearing loss, as it often does for conductive hearing loss. In this case, both thresholds and loudness tolerance would be elevated and we could simply overcome the increased impedance with amplification. If all we had to do was deliver the "lost dBs" to an intact cochlea, then we could simply match the hearing aid gain to the degree of hearing loss. For, example, a 60 dB hearing loss would be fit with a 60 dB gain hearing aid.

Most people with hearing loss, however, have sensorineural hearing losses with the *dynamic range* smaller than normal. Dynamic range is the "area" of residual hearing between the hearing thresholds (softest levels one can hear) and the uncomfortable listening levels (loudest levels one can tolerate). Consider the example of someone with mild hearing loss in the low frequencies and moderate hearing loss in the high frequencies, who has uncomfortable loudness levels of say, 100 dB HL at all audiometric frequencies. For this person, the dynamic range, the area between thresholds and loudness tolerance levels, would be larger for the low frequencies than for the high frequencies.

Most people with sensorineural hearing loss have a reduced dynamic range, with soft sounds not being audible, yet intense sounds are still heard as just as loudly as they are by those with normal hearing. It is as if the "floor" of hearing sensitivity is elevated, but the "ceiling" of loudness tolerance is unchanged. Hearing aids for someone with this type of loss must amplify soft sounds below the person's threshold by a lot; but intense sounds cannot be amplified by the same amount without dramatically exceeding the person's tolerance for loudness. More is discussed on dynamic range in Chapter 3.

Killion and Fikret-Pasa (1993) rejected the concept of "mirroring" the audiogram with full gain, but their reasons were different than those given here. They stated that mirroring the audiogram is unrealistic, because it would amplify background noise too much. Mirroring the audiogram of a person with a sensorineural hearing loss of 40 dB HL would mean giving a full 40 dB of gain for the person to hear 0 dB HL sounds. This would theoretically restore normal hearing, but the sound pressure level of most background ambient noise is about 40 to 45 dB(A). Even a person with normal hearing levels would not be able to hear audiometric pure tones softer than 20 to 25 dB HL in this common environment. A full gain of 40 dB would amplify both the ambient 40 to 45 dB(A) of background noise and the 20 to 25 dB HL pure tones buried within it. Therefore, providing a full 40 dB of gain would not do much good. It would be too much gain. Killion argued that a better gain target for the 40 dB sensorineural hearing loss would be less (e.g., around 20 to 25 dB).

Basically, we cannot use linear hearing aids which amplify all sound inputs by the same amount; if we do, we will have to choose hearing aids that offer less gain overall. This is exactly what Lybarger found by trial and error as early as the 1940s (Lybarger, 1944)!

Lybarger's Half-Gain Rule

Lybarger proposed the "half-gain" rule that seemed to work well with linear hearing aids, which were the "state-of-the art" of hearing aid technology at the time. When fitting people with full-gain hearing aids (e.g., 60 dB gain for a 60 dB HL input), he would talk to clients and ask them to turn the volume to where they liked it. They would usually turn the volume halfway up. Thus, by trial and error, Lybarger found that most people preferred about half the gain for their hearing loss (e.g., 30 dB gain for a 60 dB hearing loss). In this way, his clients could get a comfortable amount of gain for both soft and loud speech and still be able to tolerate the output. The half gain rule is a *compromise* between (1) the linear circuitry he had available at the time and (2) the reduced dynamic range of the damaged non-linear cochlea.

A Few Threshold-based Fitting Methods

The half-gain fitting method is still in use today and it forms the basis of many subsequent "threshold-based" fitting methods developed in the 1960s and 1970s. A few of the more popular "children" of the half-gain rule are: Berger's half-gain method (Berger, Hagberg, & Rane, 1980), prescription of gain and output (POGO) by McCandless (1983), the one-third gain method by Libby (1986), and the National Acoustics Lab-revised (NAL-R) by Byrne and Dillon (1986).

Threshold-based fitting methods offered an alternative to the requirements of speech testing as outlined by Carhart (1946). The required gain for threshold-based methods is determined from the thresholds and is presented as a theoretical target. The actual gain from any hearing aid is matched to the target to determine how close it comes to meeting the goal. According to McCandless & Lyregaard (1983), speech intelligibility testing was time consuming and showed a lot of statistical variability. On the other hand, a threshold-based approach with a target could more easily identify the frequency response of hearing aids. The results of hearing aid trimmer settings and changes to these settings were also more visible with threshold-based fitting methods than they would be with tests of speech discrimination and speech reception in a sound field (Libby, 1988; McCandless & Lyregaard, 1983).

Typical half-gain threshold-based fitting methods offer a single "target" of gain for any one particular hearing loss configuration, because they all assume linear hearing aid circuitry and use audiometric hearing thresholds to determine the appropriate amounts of gain. These methods assume that the target should be met with the volume control of the hearing aid set to a user setting. They also share the suggestion that the hearing aid should have about 10 to 15 dB extra or reserve gain above and beyond the user volume control setting (Libby, 1988). All the threshold fitting methods discussed here attempt to maximize the intelligibility of speech at the client's most comfortable listening level. Threshold-based fitting methods also include suggestions for determining the MPO of a hearing aid to prevent the aided gain from exceeding the client's uncomfortable listening levels (UCL).

For most threshold-based fitting methods, the gain prescribed for the lower frequencies is less than that prescribed for higher frequencies. This is done to reduce the "upward spread of masking" (see Chapter 1). One of the main complaints of hearing aid wearers is that of amplified background noise competing with amplified speech. Background noise consists of many frequencies. Colloquial clinical knowledge has it that the "hubbub" of background speech noise is mostly low-frequency energy, while the mid-to-high frequencies contribute more weight to the intelligibility of speech. Because low frequencies mask high frequencies better than highs mask lows, amplified background noise may indeed wreak havoc with speech intelligibility, especially for those who wear hearing aids.

It is interesting to note, however, that for any particular hearing loss, the targets suggested by threshold-based fitting methods are all markedly different, as shown in Figure 2–6.

The Berger half-gain fitting method surfaced earlier than the others. For the hearing loss in Figure 2–4, the Berger fitting method offers the most gain at 1000 and 2000 Hz. For this fitting method, the most important speech cues for optimal understanding were believed to be at these particular frequency regions. Therefore, more than 1/2 gain was offered for 1000 Hz and 2000 Hz. Less than 1/2 gain was offered for the low frequencies to optimize speech intelligibility and reduce the upward spread of masking. To arrive at the specific gain requirements for a particular hearing loss, Berger suggested the following: multiply the hearing loss at 250 Hz by .45, at 500 Hz by .50, at 1000 Hz by .625, at 2000 Hz by .667, at 3000 Hz by .588, at 4000 Hz by .50. These multiplication values represented the various weights of importance

A Comparison of Threshold Methods

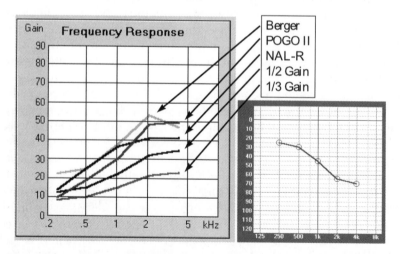

Figure 2–6. Five different threshold-based fitting methods give five different targets for the same person's hearing loss. There is even one more complication: the differences between the targets, themselves, vary with different hearing losses!

for speech intelligibility that Berger attached to each audiometric frequency. Berger recommended a reserve gain of 10 dB. To calculate maximum power output, Berger converted uncomfortable listening levels (measured in a sound field) to units of dB SPL, and then setting the MPO 4 to 6 dB above this level (Berger, Hagberg, & Rane, 1980).

The POGO method came into use after the Berger method. For the hearing loss in Figure 2–4, POGO asks for about as much high-frequency (4000 Hz) gain as Berger's method. The POGO method is quite straightforward in its calculations: it asks for exactly one-half gain at each audiometric frequency (multiply each threshold by .50), with less than one-half gain for the low frequencies of 250 Hz (10 dB less) and 500 Hz (5 dB less). The Berger and POGO fitting method give similar weight to the high frequencies, because these frequencies are thought to contribute greatly to speech intelligibility. However, POGO proposes considerably less gain for the mid and low frequencies than than Berger method, in order to further reduce the possibility of the upward spread of masking. Like the Berger method, a 10 dB reserve gain is also suggested by POGO. McCandless & Lyregaard (1983) note that a reason for some hearing aid rejections was that of exceeding uncomfortable loudness levels with the hearing aid gain requirements. Accordingly, the maximum power output is another parameter of concern for POGO. Unlike the Berger method, POGO suggests that the MPO on the hearing aid should be set to the client's UCL as measured in dB hearing level (HL). A POGO II method was later developed for more severe hearing losses.

The Libby 1/3–2/3 gain fitting method is similar to that of POGO, except that for those with mild-to-moderately severe hearing losses, the thresholds at each audiometric test frequency are multiplied by 1/3. According to Libby (1986), these clients and those with precipitous high-frequency hearing losses, do not actually wear their hearing aids at a volume that provides 1/2 gain for their hearing losses. On the contrary, these clients tend to prefer a volume setting that reflects a gain closer to 1/3 of their thresholds. Like the Berger and POGO methods, Libby suggests less gain for the low frequencies of 250 Hz and 500 Hz. Perhaps because of the reduced overall gain suggested by the 1/3 gain method, Libby recommended a reduction of only 5 dB from 1/3 gain at 250 Hz and 3 dB from 1/3 gain at 500 Hz. For severe and profound hearing losses, Libby recommended a 2/3 gain rule, because he found these people to prefer more gain.

The NAL-R fitting method seems to have surfaced in popularity later than the other methods mentioned, and in the author's experience, it is the most popular of the threshold-based fitting methods today. The main focus of NAL-R method is to amplify the frequencies of unaided speech so that they sound equally loud at a comfortable listening level and maximize intelligibility of speech for people with hearing loss. The original NAL fitting method (Byrne & Tonnison, 1976) was subsequently found not to consistently accomplish this objective and so the NAL method was revised (Byrne & Dillon, 1983)-hence, the NAL-R fitting method. For a flat audiogram, NAL-R suggests about 10 dB more gain at 500 Hz and about 3–4 dB more gain at 3000 Hz and 4000 Hz than the original NAL fitting method.

In general, for any particular hearing loss, NAL-R suggests slightly less than 1/2 gain. The NAL-R method also tries to prevent excessive high-frequency gain for clients with steeply sloping hearing losses. It requires a more complex calculation than the other mentioned fitting methods to determine the appropriate gain. The calculation has three elements: (1) a constant value, with the average thresholds of 500 Hz, 1000 Hz, and 2000 Hz multiplied by .05; (2) thresholds at each audiometric frequency threshold are multiplied by .31; and (3) different gain values for each frequency required to make various frequency regions of speech sound equally loud. As to the third element in the NAL-R calculation, the low frequencies are given less gain than the mid frequencies (e.g., −17 dB for 250 Hz), and the high frequencies are given slightly less gain than the mid frequencies (e.g., −2 dB for 4000 Hz). These three elements must be added together to determine the prescribed gain for each audiometric frequency. For more explanation or specifics, the reader is encouraged to read the original NAL-R article by Byrne & Dillon (1986).

In general, the NAL-R fitting method also suggests a "flatter" gain than the other methods. Figure 2–4 shows that the gain proposed by the NAL-R fitting method is less than POGO for the high frequencies and more than POGO for the low frequencies. Compared to Berger, the suggested gain for NAL-R is similar for 500 and 1000 Hz, but is less at 2000 Hz and higher. The NAL-R fitting method suggests a 15 dB reserve gain above the client's user volume control setting. There is now a version of NAL, called the NAL-NL1 (which stands for Non-linear, version 1), which is based on compression hearing aids; this is discussed further in Chapter 3.

It should be reiterated that all of the threshold-based fitting methods briefly described here provide a *single* target for any one particular audiometric hearing loss configuration, because they assume linear amplification (which provides the same gain for all input sound levels). Each method acknowledges that the most common type of hearing loss is sensorineural in nature, and, also, that although soft sounds are inaudible, intense sounds may still be heard as loud as they would for normal hearing. The result of this phenomenon is a reduced dynamic range. The target for any particular hearing loss and for any particular threshold-based fitting method arises out of a *compromise* between the reduced dynamic range encountered with sensorineural hearing loss and linear hearing aid technology.

SUMMARY

■ Unlike optometry, there is no single, universally accepted hearing aid fitting method; that is, the fitting is not necessarily done "correctly" or "incorrectly." Every few years, old fitting methods seem to be replaced by new ones.

■ Simply "mirroring" the audiogram with full linear gain is impossible, because for those with sensorineural hearing loss, the "floor" of hearing sensitivity may be elevated compared to normal hearing, but their "ceiling" of loudness tolerance is similar to those with normal hearing. The half-gain method of Lybarger arose out of a compromise between (1) the linear technology available at the time and (2) the nonlinear function of the cochlea.

■ Many of the threshold-based fitting methods were derived from the half-gain fitting method. These methods assume linear circuitry. They all focus on audiometric thresholds, and acknowledge a reduced dynamic range with sensorineural hearing loss, but they do not focus specifically on loudness growth. Loudness growth and some newer fitting methods will be discussed in Chapter 3.

RECOMMENDED READING

Killion, M. C. (1997). The SIN report: Circuits haven't solved the hearing-in-noise problem. *The Hearing Journal, 50*(10), 28-34.

McCandless, G. A. (1994). Overview and rationale of threshold-based hearing aid selection procedures. In M. Valente (Ed.), *Strategies for selecting and verifying hearing aid fittings* (pp. 1-18). New York: Thieme Medical Publishers, Inc.

Preves, D. (1997, July). Directional microphone use in ITE hearing instruments. *The Hearing Review, 4*(7), 21-27.

CHAPTER 3

Loudness Growth and Fitting Considerations

In this chapter, the psychoacoustic concepts of normal versus abnormal loudness growth and three of the newer hearing aid fitting methods are discussed. Lately, it seems that we are hearing a lot about loudness growth. Loudness growth occurs from one's hearing thresholds, with perceptions of sounds ranging from "just barely audible" up to the loudest sounds that one can tolerate. New hearing aid fitting methods focus on the "area" or *dynamic range* that lies between these two extremes, namely: uncomfortable loudness (UCL) or threshold of discomfort (TD), minus speech reception threshold (SRT), or pure-tone thresholds.

A typical dynamic range is about 100 dB, where the thresholds are close to 0 dB HL and the UCL or TD is at around 100 dB. For people with this dynamic range, a 50 dB HL sound might be perceived as "comfortable" in loudness. For a mild-to-moderate sensorineural hearing loss, such as presbycusis, however, a 50 dB HL sound might be barely audible, whereas the UCL or TD will still be at around 100 dB HL. In this case, the dynamic range is smaller (50 dB) and loudness "grows" much faster that it does for the normal-hearing person with the wider 100 dB dynamic range. Compared to someone with normal hearing, the "floor" of hearing sensitivity is elevated for the person with the sensorineural hearing loss; on the other hand, the "ceiling" of loudness tolerance is about the same as it is for someone with normal hearing.

Many clinicians want to restore normal loudness growth for their clients. There are sounds in our environment that unaided, normally hearing persons perceive as "soft," "comfortable," and "loud." Ideally, for persons with hearing loss who wear hearing aids, these sounds should be perceived the same way. If this objective is accomplished with hearing aids, then normal loudness growth has been restored for the client. In the example of the person with mild-to-moderate sensorineural hearing loss, restoring normal loudness growth may require a hearing aid that provides very different gain for soft input sounds (such as 20 dB HL) than it does for more intense input sounds (such as 80 dB HL). Only a *compression* hearing aid can accomplish this objective.

As discussed in Chapter 2, linear hearing aids provide the same gain for different input sound levels. Fitting methods that generate a single target of gain for a particular hearing loss assume linear amplification, because the target is applicable for any input sound level of intensity. Such fitting methods are the threshold-based methods discussed in Chapter 2. However, the gain for *different* input levels is not specifically addressed by these methods.

A new set of fitting methods has recently emerged and is rapidly gaining in popularity; these are often known as "suprathreshold" fitting methods. Suprathreshold fitting methods provide more than one target, where each target represents a different amount of gain (or output) that is prescribed for different input sound levels of intensity. In this way, compression is specifically addressed by the newer, suprathreshold fitting methods.

Suprathreshold fitting methods assume the reality and ever-increasing presence of nonlinear (compression circuitry) in hearing aids. Today's hearing aids mostly use compression and many different types of compression are discussed specifically in Chapter 4. Some types of compression are especially effective at limiting the output to not exceed one's UCL or TD. On the other hand, there are some types of compression where the specific goal is to shrink a normal (large) dynamic range into a smaller range that occurs with sensorineural hearing loss. No one compression can be said to be "better" than another; the choice of compression for any particular case depends on the clinical objective and what type might be best for the client.

In this chapter, the three concepts of loudness growth, new fitting methods, and compression are discussed together: (1) abnormal loudness growth is the problem the person with hearing loss takes to the clinician; (2) the newer fitting methods set the particular goals for amplification, based on the client's hearing loss and; (3) the various types of compression in hearing aids are the ways or means whereby to accomplish the goals that are set out by the fitting methods.

LOUDNESS GROWTH

As mentioned in Chapter 1, hearing aids cannot replace the internal function of the cochlea with its active traveling wave and mechanically mobile outer hair cells (OHCs). But we are making small steps toward this goal. Figure 3–1 shows what present hearing aid technology *can* do to imitate the function of the OHCs for mild-to-moderate sensorineural hearing loss (SNHL); namely, help restore normal loudness growth. Note in the figure, the horizontal axis represents the physical world of intensity and the vertical axis represents the corresponding psychoacoustic perception of loudness.

SNHL usually exhibits a reduced dynamic range. The normal-hearing person in Figure 3-1 has a dynamic range of 90 dB, which means that 0 dB HL sounds are perceived as "just barely audible" and

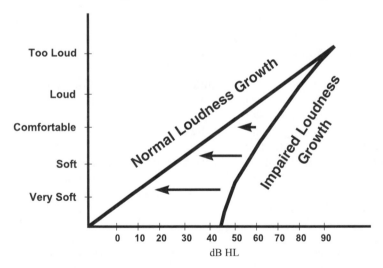

Figure 3–1. The goal of amplification for mild-to-moderate sensorineural hearing loss is to restore normal loudness growth. The X axis shows the physical dimension of increasing input sound intensity to the hearing aid. The Y axis shows corresponding psychoacoustic dimension of increased loudness perception. We don't know how to sharpen a traveling wave with hearing aids, yet. But we *can* amplify soft sounds more than loud sounds. To do this, a hearing aid should amplify soft sounds by a lot, and loud sounds by little or nothing at all.

90 dB HL sounds are perceived as "too loud." For the hearing loss, the dynamic range is only 45 dB, because the threshold (for some particular frequency) is 45 dB HL and the uncomfortable loudness level is 90 dB HL. Note that 90 dB is perceived as "too loud" for both the normal-hearing person and the person with mild-to-moderate SNHL. The difference for the two populations is mainly for perception of low-intensity sounds. The loudness growth is more rapid or steep for the person with the SNHL than it is for those with normal hearing. It is as if the "ceiling" is the same with both normal hearing and with hearing loss, but the "floor" is elevated with the hearing loss.

What should a hearing aid do in this situation to best imitate the function of the outer hair cells? It should restore normal loudness growth. To do this, soft sounds need to be amplified by a lot, and loud sounds should be amplified by little or nothing at all. At high intensities, the role of the hearing aid should "disappear" or according to Killion (1997c) it should become acoustically "transparent." The cochlea is a nonlinear organ; just because thresholds increase does not mean that loudness tolerance levels increase as well. Accordingly, we should provide nonlinear gain with hearing aids so that low-intensity input sounds are amplified by more than high-intensity input sounds.

There is one thing missing from Figure 3–1; namely, frequency. Figure 3–2 shows three dimensions: (1) intensity in dB sound pressure level (SPL), (2) frequency in hertz (Hz), and (3) loudness growth curves (sometimes called "equal loudness contours," "Fletcher-Munsen curves," or "phon" curves). In addition, the loudness growth for normal hearing and for a typical mild-to-moderate SNHL is compared.

The lighter curves, or contours, show equal loudness perceptions for normal hearing across the frequency range. Along any one particular curve, each frequency along the bottom axis sounds equally loud to normal ears; note that each frequency requires a different SPL to be perceived as equally loud. This difference in required SPL is especially evident for the lower curves representing softer sounds.

The bottom-most curve is closest to what is known as 0 dB hearing level (HL). Sometimes called the "minimal audibility curve," this bottom contour represents the perception of "just barely audible" by normal listeners and it shows that our best hearing is somewhere between 1000 and 5000 Hz. To be just barely audible, the low frequencies and extreme high frequencies need to be more intense than the mid frequencies. At high intensities such as 100 dB SPL, the curves flatten out, which means that for high intensities, there is less difference in SPL required for us to judge the sounds at all the frequencies as being equally loud. Here it becomes evident once again, that the cochlea is a nonlinear organ; that is, the cochlea works differently with soft sound inputs than it does for intense sounds.

The shape of the bottom-most curves has a lot to do with why we have a "loudness" switch on our stereo or why on equalizers the buttons are often arranged like a "smile." At low-volume control settings, we need an extra boost for some frequencies to hear all the frequencies equally loud. At high volume settings, however, the equal loudness lines flatten out. This means that for intense sounds we no longer need as great a difference in sound pressure levels across the frequency range to hear all the frequencies equally loud and this is why we then turn the loudness switch off.

For normal hearing, there is a normal spread of the curves or loudness contours. Note that the dynamic range, or area, between the top and bottom curves in Figure 3–2 is largest for the mid frequencies and smallest for the very low frequencies. A small dynamic range implies a "fast" loudness "growth." The smaller dynamic range for the low frequencies means that the growth of loudness from sensations of "just barely audible" to "very loud" grow relatively fast for the low frequencies and more slowly for the mid frequencies.

With SNHL:
The "Ceiling" is the Same, but the "Floor" is Raised

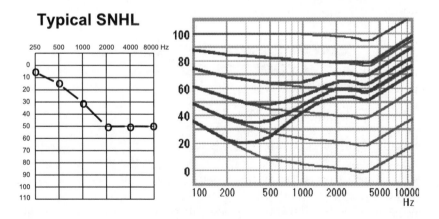

Figure 3–2. Frequency, intensity, and loudness growth are shown together in one graph. Here we can see that for mild-to-moderate sensorineural hearing loss (darker lines), the "ceiling" of loudness tolerance is the same as it is for normal hearing; it is the "floor" of hearing sensitivity that becomes elevated for the hearing loss. The cochlea is indeed a nonlinear organ.

The equal loudness contours for normal hearing show a normal dynamic range of up to about 100 dB. For the SNHL (the darker curves in Figure 3–2), the bottom curves become elevated for the mid to high frequencies. On the other hand, the top curves for hearing loss are similar to those for normal hearing. The curves for the hearing loss are squeezed, or pinched, together in the mid to high frequencies, which shows a smaller dynamic range. For these high frequencies, the person with SNHL cannot hear soft sounds. Yet high-intensity sounds are heard just as loudly as they are by people with normal hearing. Once again, for the person with normal hearing and the person with SNHL, the "ceiling" is the same; it is the "floor" that is elevated for the person with hearing loss. Loudness growth is more rapid for the high frequencies where the ceiling and the floor are closest together.

It could and perhaps *should* be asked as to why these curves exist in the first place. Why does the human minimal audibility curve (the bottom-most curve) show differences in hearing sensitivity in the first place? The difference in normal hearing sensitivity is largely caused by the physical properties of the middle ear and, to a lesser extent, the outer ear (Durrant & Lovrinic, 1984). As a system of physical structures, the middle ear has its own sum total characteristic properties of mass and stiffness, and thus has its own resonances that pass some frequencies through more easily than others. In short, the middle ear is not as efficient at passing some frequencies as it is at others. The resonances of the concha (4000 to 5000 Hz) and outer ear canal (around 2700 Hz) also contribute to the shape of the human minimal audibility curve.

COMPRESSION AND NORMAL LOUDNESS GROWTH

Recall from Chapter 2 the basic hearing aid formula: *input* plus *gain* equals *output*. Linear hearing aids give the same gain for all input levels, and threshold-based fitting methods that assume linear amplification offer a single target for gain, which is based on the thresholds of the hearing loss. Because the gain is the same for all input intensity levels in linear circuits, there is no need for more than one target. For high-intensity input sounds, a linear hearing aid with a lot of gain will give an output that may exceed one's uncomfortable loudness levels and so the maximum output is "clipped," which may result in distorted sound quality.

For compression hearing aids, a single target for gain no longer tells the whole story, because compression circuits provide different amounts of gain for different input levels. Compression tends to cut down or reduce the gain as the input levels increase, but this should not be done at the expense of making the *outputs* all the same. The output for each input level is important to consider, because the output is the real result or "goods" that reaches the ear of the person wearing the hearing aid. If the gain goes down as much as the inputs go up, then the outputs will all sound equally loud and the person wearing the hearing aid will not be able to tell when things are actually getting louder in the real world.

Most gain should be given to soft input sounds, so the person with hearing loss can hear the sounds. For example, a person with a 60 decibel (dB) hearing loss trying to listen to 1 or 2 dB hearing level (HL) sounds should in theory be given 60 dB of gain. As the inputs increase in intensity, the gain should go down, but not quite as much as the amount by which the inputs increase. The outputs will then still increase with input level, but not by as much as the inputs increase. In this way, persons with hearing loss still experience a growth of loudness for sounds as they naturally occur in the environment. Thus, a normally large dynamic range will be "shrunk" into a smaller one (more on this topic will be covered in Chapter 4).

Newer fitting methods that address compression hearing aids specify the desired gain or output for several input levels (e.g., soft, medium, and loud inputs). As clinicians, we often see advertisements for certain compression hearing aids where the stated goal is to "restore normal loudness growth" for the client who demonstrates "abnormal" loudness growth. Indeed, many nonlinear (or compression) hearing aids are specifically designed to "restore normal loudness growth" for the person who has sensorineural hearing loss and a smaller-than-normal dynamic range.

SUPRATHRESHOLD FITTING METHODS, COMPRESSION, AND LOUDNESS GROWTH

From the late 1980s to the present, we have become enamored with suprathreshold fitting methods that assume compression in hearing aids, specifically intended to address the reduced dynamic range for those with SNHL. Three new fitting methods are briefly discussed in this chapter. Each fitting method has a different slant. But because they are all concerned with the dynamic range and loudness growth in some way, they are often called "suprathreshold" fitting methods.

Fig6 Fitting Method

The name "Fig6" actually comes from Figure 6 in an article written by Killion (1993), describing the principles of this method. This method is mentioned first because, for the clinician learning new fitting methods, it is a "bridge" between the older threshold-based methods that assume linear hearing aids and the newer suprathreshold-based methods which do not. The gain graph of Fig6, in terms of amplitude and frequency axes, is laid out the same way as those of the earlier threshold-based methods. In addition, along with its own three targets, Fig6 also includes the NAL-R target, which allows for an instant visual comparison. These attributes make the "mental leap" from past methods to Fig6 smaller or easier than for the other two methods described here.

The Fig6 fitting method employs a computer program that calculates the gain needed for any particular hearing loss. The calculated gain by the Fig6 computer program is based on *average* loudness growth data taken from several studies that demonstrate how the loudness growth for SNHL compares to that for normal hearing (Gitles & Tillman-Niquette, 1995). Because Fig6 is based on average loudness growth, it requires no loudness perception testing beyond the standard audiogram, an aspect that is attractive to many clinicians. This enables a relatively quick fitting process, because it eliminates the need to measure the loudness growth on each client being fit with hearing aids.

The measurement of loudness growth is relatively subjective compared to that of behavioral pure-tone threshold audiometry. Consequently, measures of perceptions of "soft but audible," "comfortable," "loud but not too loud," and so on, can differ from person to person, can differ within a given client from day-to-day, and can differ with instructions provided from examiner to examiner. Furthermore, loudness growth, if measured at all thoroughly, should be assessed at more than one frequency because, as we have seen from the previous discussion on equal loudness contours, loudness may "grow" more rapidly at some frequencies than at others.

The Fig6 method is intended to be used especially with hearing aids that have "wide dynamic range compression" circuitry (discussed specifically in Chapter 4). The idea behind this type of compression and the Fig6 fitting method, in general, is to deliver incoming soft-intensity, medium-intensity, and high-intensity sounds to the listener in such a way that they are respectively heard as "soft," "medium," and "loud." In other words, the goal is to shrink a normally wide dynamic range into one that is smaller. This goal is kept in mind with knowledge of normal versus abnormal loudness growth; namely, that for most people with SNHL, the "ceiling" of loudness tolerance is changed very little from normal-it is the "floor" that is elevated the most.

When discussing the principles behind Fig6, Killion (1993) rejected the concept of "mirroring" the audiogram with full gain, even for very soft input intensity levels (as noted in Chapter 2). The Fig6 fitting method thus provides less than full gain for soft input intensity levels and then decreases the gain as the input intensity levels increase.

Fig6 has three targets for three different input intensity levels, instead of having a single target for a single amount of gain (see Figure 3–3). Each target represents the amount of gain needed that is based on the specific hearing loss on the bottom right corner of the figure. The bottom-most curve or function represents the amount of gain needed for high-intensity (95 dB SPL) input levels (note that it provides little or none for the lower frequency sounds that are more intense in typical conversational speech). The middle-most function represents the gain needed for moderate (65 dB SPL) input levels (more gain is provided for the high-frequency sounds). The top function represents the gain for soft (40 dB SPL) input levels (note that the most gain is provided for these

Fig6. Fitting Formula

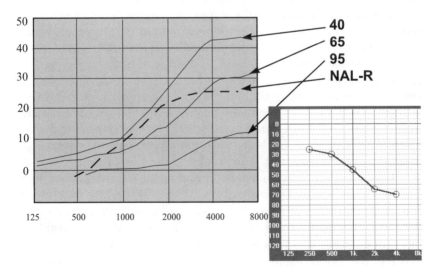

Figure 3–3. The Fig6 fitting method has three gain targets and also shows the NAL-R target. All targets are based on the same hearing loss.

softer high-frequency sounds). The Fig6 fitting method assumes the use of compression hearing aids because nonlinear (compression) hearing aids automatically reduce their gain for increased input sound intensity levels. As one can see, the prescribed gain goes down as the input intensity goes up.

The particular input levels used in Fig6 were chosen to represent different levels of conversational speech (Gitles & Tillman-Niquette, 1995). The input of 40 dB SPL (around 20 dB HL) approximates the least intense elements of typical conversational speech, although the input of 65 dB SPL (around 50 dB HL) approaches that of usual, ongoing conversational speech, and the 95 dB SPL input is more representative of levels for loud music and speech. Recall that typical speech fluctuates from about 35 dB SPL for soft consonant sounds to about 75 dB SPL for loud vowel sounds. It is interesting to note some differences between the targets for Fig6 and NAL-R that are displayed on the Fig6 fitting screen (see Figure 3–3). For the typical mild-to-moderate SNHL, Fig6 provides more high-frequency emphasis and less mid-frequency emphasis than the NAL-R method.

The Fig6 method also addresses issues such as (1) the real-ear-to-coupler-difference (RECD) and (2) the microphone placement on different styles of hearing aids. Both of these measures are important to consider, because they each affect the sound output from the hearing aid that reaches the eardrum. RECD is a measure of how the resonance of an individual real ear canal is different from that of the standard 2cc artificial coupler used to measure hearing aid performance. The output from the receiver of the hearing aid is "sculpted" by the particular resonance of any individual's real ear canal and these changes alter the sound from the 2-cc coupler output that is given on hearing aid specification sheets.

Microphone placements on BTE, ITE, and completely-in-canal (CIC) hearing aids are all different relative to the side of the head, the shape of the concha of the pinna, and so on. The sound input to the microphone of a hearing aid also is "sculpted" by its immediate surroundings, and this altered input, when added to the gain of the hearing aid will have an effect on the eventual output to the eardrum. The microphone located on the faceplate of a CIC hearing aid, for example, is buried deep inside the canal; the concha is left relatively unoccluded with a CIC compared to full concha shell ITE hearing aid. The sound going into the CIC microphone is, therefore, more affected by the resonance of the concha than that of the full-concha ITE. The clinician who wants to arrive at a truer estimation of hearing aid output would do well to consider the factors of RECD and microphone placement.

IHAFF Fitting Method

The name IHAFF stands for the Independent Hearing Aid Fitting Forum, a group of 12 audiologists who first got together in 1993 to devise a fitting method that would help clinicians determine appropriate compression characteristics to best meet the needs of their clients. Many different types of compression with many different options were being developed and offered by hearing aid manufacturers. On the other hand, appropriate fitting methods that could guide clinicians in choosing optimal compression characteristics for a client were not available. It was out of frustration with this situation that IHAFF was established.

The basic idea behind IHAFF is to choose the type of compression circuit that will best restore a particular client's *individual* loudness growth to normal all across the audiometric frequency range. The IHAFF method tries to provide a nexus between actual environmental sounds and the perception of those sounds by the aided listener who has hearing loss. Sounds that are soft to the person with normal hearing should still sound soft to the listener with hearing aids; sounds that are comfortable for the person with normal hearing ought to sound the same for the listener with hearing aids, and so on (Cox, 1995).

The IHAFF fitting method relies on measured loudness growth data obtained from each individual client, because clients who have the same sensorineural hearing loss may well have different perceptions of loudness growth across the frequencies. To obtain repeatable measures from client to client, from the same client on one day to the next, and from clinic to clinic, a reliable loudness measurement tool had to be developed. As a result, the IHAFF developed the Contour Test.

The Contour Test can be implemented and scored manually or with computer software interfaced to an audiometer. The IHAFF proponents realize that to be clinically feasible, the loudness growth for every client cannot be measured at each frequency because this would require far too much time (Cox, 1995). Therefore, they recommend that loudness measurements be conducted for at least two frequencies (e.g., 500 Hz and 3000 Hz). With experience, loudness growth measurement can be obtained in about five minutes per frequency. Testing two frequencies for each ear translates into about 20 minutes of test time (Cox, 1995).

The Contour Test uses seven different loudness categories: (1) very soft, (2) soft, (3) comfortable but slightly soft, (4) comfortable, (5) comfortable but slightly loud, (6) loud but okay, and (7) uncomfortably loud. These loudness levels are used to find corresponding intensity levels for pulsed warble tones (as opposed to steady pure tones). Pulsed warble tones are used because they are narrow in bandwidth and are thus, good for determining hearing aid frequency characteristics (Cox, Alexander, Taylor, & Gray, 1997). Furthermore, present audiometers can easily produce warble tones.

Because speech signals, rather than warble tones, however, are the primary input sounds of interest to most listeners, the goal of the IHAFF method is to restore normal loudness for speech. According to the IHAFF method, soft speech is about 50 dB SPL, average speech is about 65 dB SPL, and loud speech is about 85 dB SPL (Cox, 1995). Note that these levels differ slightly from those used with Fig6. The IHAFF fitting method attempts to position the loudness judgments for speech and warble tones *in the same relationship* as they are found in those with normal hearing. To do this, the seven loudness categories of the Contour Test are condensed into the three loudness categories of speech.

For those with normal hearing, loudness judgments for speech do not neatly correspond with loudness judgments for pulsed warble tones. To be judged as being as loud as speech, warble tones have to be more intense in dB SPL. For example "loud" speech is similar to "comfortable" warble tones; and both "average" and "soft" speech fall within the range of "soft" warble tones.

When actually using the IHAFF fitting method, clients with hearing loss first complete the Contour Test, allowing clinicians to determine their loudness judgments across the frequency and intensity ranges for the pulsed warble tones. These will, of course, be different from normal. The typical "soft," "average," and "loud" levels of speech input are then repositioned (by the computer software) to be relative to the areas of loudness judgment for the warble tones, just as they are for normal hearing. The resulting amount of gain prescribed is derived from the "distance" between the three "normal" speech levels and the three "repositioned" speech levels for a client with hearing loss. Ultimately, one type of compression or another will be prescribed, because the gain will differ for each of the three different speech input levels. Cox (1995) pointed out that the required gain should change with input intensity level and with frequency, because persons with high-frequency SNHL will have especially narrow dynamic ranges for the high frequencies.

Once loudness growth testing is completed via the Contour Test, the results can be entered on the visual input/output locator algorithm (VIOLA) to determine the compression characteristics that will best accommodate the changing gain requirements. Figure 3–4 shows two VIOLA graphs that typically appear on the computer screen, one for a lower frequency (e.g., 500 Hz) and the other for a higher frequency (e.g., 3000 Hz). Each graph shows input intensity level on the X axis

IHAFF

TEST	500 #1	500 #2	500 #3	3000 #1	3000 #2	3000 #3
Gain at 40 dB						
Comp Threshold 1						
Comp. Ratio 1						
Comp. Threshold 2						
Comp. Ratio 1						
Max. Output						

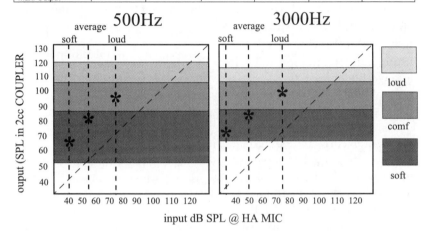

Figure 3–4. The IHAFF fitting method uses the VIOLA (visual input/output locator algorithm) program that shows input/output graphs for any two selected frequencies. The above example is based on a person with mild-to-moderate SNHL and the two selected frequencies are 500 and 3000 Hz. Up to three different hearing aids can be compared (top). The functions (lines on the graph) for linear hearing aids and those for various types of compression hearing aids would be distinct from each other. The main idea of IHAFF is to match the gain of the hearing aid as closely as possible to the three dots for both 500 Hz and 3000 Hz

and output intensity along the Y axis. Gain is of course, the difference between input and output. A diagonal line cross each graph from the lower left corner to the top right corner represents 0 dB of gain.

In the background of each graph, three horizontal shaded areas represent the ranges of loudness judgment for the warble tones from the Contour Test. Recall that the seven loudness categories for warble tones are condensed into three loudness categories for speech. For each graph, three vertical lines called "soft," "average," and "loud" represent the typical unaided speech levels for each frequency, as mentioned earlier. Each graph also shows three asterisks, which are positioned along the vertical lines. These represent the IHAFF targets: namely, the gain required to amplify soft, average, and loud input speech.

Unaided "soft," "average," and "loud" speech does not change from client to client; therefore, these vertical lines are consistently placed relative to any particular frequency chosen. Because of the relationship between loudness judgements for warble tones and speech, the asterisks are always placed in the same position relative to the horizontal shaded background loudness areas. The shaded areas, however, will differ for each client, depending on his or her own particular loudness judgments. The distance between each asterisk and the diagonal line represents the gain required by IHAFF.

Figure 3–4 shows the VIOLA graphs for a mild-to-moderate SNHL. The hearing for the high frequencies is worse than that for the low frequencies; as a result, the dynamic range for the high frequencies is smaller than that for the low frequencies. Note that the horizontal shaded areas are bunched closer together for 3000 Hz than they are for 500 Hz. Looking at the distance from the diagonal (0 dB gain) line to the asterisks for each graph, it can be seen that the prescribed gain for soft input speech is about 25 dB for 500 Hz, and about 30 to 35 dB for 3000 Hz. For loud input speech, the prescribed gain is about 25 dB for 500 Hz, and about 30 dB for 3000 Hz.

The strength of the VIOLA program and IHAFF, in general, is that it allows the clinician to instantly visualize the varying processing schemes of different hearing aids. For example, a linear hearing aid can be compared to various types of compression hearing aids and the results can be compared to see which circuit characteristics will best match the VIOLA targets. The IHAFF approach, like the Fig6 method also includes considerations for RECD and microphone placements.

The clinician can specify gain and output characteristics to see which combination will best match the targets for each graph (see Figure 3–4). Two "threshold kneepoints" and two "compression ratios" can be specified (these terms will be described in Chapter 4). From hearing aid specifications, a hearing aid can then be chosen to fit the client, based on the IHAFF approach.

The Abbreviated Profile of Hearing Aid Benefit (APHAB) is included as part of the IHAFF protocol. This 24-item questionnaire quantifies the qualitative psychosocial benefits for the client who wears the hearing aids and compares the client's results to previously gathered normative data (Cox & Alexander, 1995). The IHAFF approach is sometimes referred to as the "IHAFF suite" because it advises the use of (1) the Contour Test, (2) the VIOLA, and (3) the APHAB.

Some clinicians may fault IHAFF for requiring measured loudness growth that is more time consuming than using averaged data. Furthermore, most compression hearing aids currently do not possess two threshold kneepoints and two different compression ratios. Finally, despite the best efforts of the clinician, the chosen hearing aid candidates may not at all match the VIOLA targets. Van Vliet (1997) advised clinicians to choose the hearing aid that *most* matches the target, even if it does not look like a tight fit or a close match. The IHAFF approach, in general, does highlight the original concern of the group that founded it: There is a great chasm between the state-of-the-art hearing aid technology and that which the newer fitting methods require.

DSL Fitting Method

The desired sensation level (DSL) fitting method began out of concern for the fitting requirements of the pediatric population, but its use has also been generalized to adults (Seewald, 1997). The development of oral speech and language depends first and foremost on the *audibility* or ability to hear all of the sounds of speech. This is especially important for children who develop their hearing loss before or during speech and language acquisition. The DSL fitting method is an attempt to make the sounds of speech audible for such children.

Figure 3–5 shows the spectrum of speech superimposed on an audiogram. The vowels are relatively high in intensity and low in frequency (i.e., loud sounds) compared to the unvoiced consonants, which are higher in frequency and lower in intensity (i.e., soft sounds). In the big picture of speech reception, the vowels tell us *that* we hear speech. Every word contains at least one vowel. Our discrimination of *what* word we hear, however, depends heavily on the audibility of vowel/consonant sound combinations.

To this end, the main goal of DSL is the *audibility* of speech. To make as much use of residual hearing as possible, the entire unaided speech spectrum must be amplified to fit above the hearing thresholds and yet below the loudness discomfort levels (i.e., within the dynamic range) of the person with hearing loss. Furthermore, the amplified speech spectrum must be as comfortable and undistorted as possible.

For the DSL fitting method, the input signal of speech is represented by the unaided long-term average speech spectrum (LTASS). The LTASS measurements for DSL were derived using a microphone placed at the ear level of a child (Cornelisse, Seewald, & Jamieson, 1994) rather than the customary placement of the microphone in front of a subject (Cox & Moore, 1988). As a result, the DSL group found that the LTASS consisted of relatively more low-frequency energy (close to 70 dB SPL) and less high-frequency energy than the measurements by Cox and Moore (1988). It is also important for children to hear their own voice production of high-frequency consonants to properly acquire speech (Cornelisse, Gagne, & Seewald, 1991). Because of these considerations, the DSL fitting method advocates more high-frequency output than most other fitting methods.

Speech Sounds on an Audiogram

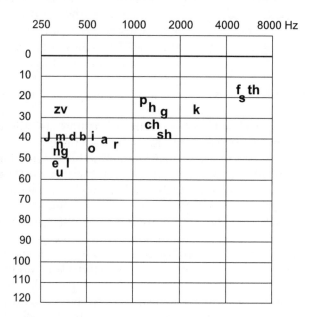

Figure 3–5. The slope of the energy present in speech rises from left to right on the typical audiogram. The vowels are more intense and lower in frequency compared to most consonants, especially the unvoiced consonants such as /s/, /f/, /th/, etc. For someone with high-frequency hearing loss, the unvoiced consonants will be especially hard to hear. Thus, the high-frequency speech sounds will obviously need to be amplified the most to make them audible.

The DSL fitting method insists on very solid foundations of measurement to ensure the validity and reliability of the hearing aid fitting. Validity of the hearing aid fitting demands that the input is really what we think it is; only then can we have a good idea about the output from the hearing aid. A more colloquial saying from some proponents of DSL is, "garbage in, garbage out." Reliability of the fitting method means that it will consistently provide the same results again and again.

The DSL fitting method attempts to account for all possible acoustic transforms that occur, beginning with the headphones used in the typical hearing test, to the standard 2cc coupler used to measure hearing aid performance, to the actual aided SPL that is delivered to the real ear of the client with the hearing aid. For example, are the audiometric pure-tone test results really what the dial reading on the audiometer says they are? If the person was tested with circumaural head-phones, calibrated on a 6cc coupler, then there is a lot of room for individual differences in the actual SPL that reaches the eardrum at each test frequency. The actual SPL delivered to the eardrum of the person might be very different from the dial reading on the audiometer for any test frequency. The real-ear-to-dial difference (REDD) thus has to be calculated across the frequency range. If this is not possible, DSL allows for average REDD values to be entered in subsequent computer target estimations. Insert headphones, on the other hand, allow less room for variability and are recommended. Furthermore, they are calibrated on a 2cc coupler like hearing aids and are, therefore, preferred.

Loudness tolerance levels or UCLs can also be measured individually on clients and then entered on the DSL computer software. Average values for UCLs across the frequency range can also be chosen to speed up the fitting process.

The style of hearing aid is also important to DSL, because as already mentioned, it determines the microphone location and, hence the typical ear canal resonances that can come into play. Similar to the Fig6 and IHAFF fitting methods, this is information that the DSL computer fitting program requires.

The RECD (see Fig6) is of central concern to DSL, as it is to the Fig6 and IHAFF fitting methods. The Audioscan™ and Frye™ hearing aid test systems are examples of test equipment that include software for the DSL fitting method. Such systems employ a unique input signal, a "dynamic" speech sound stimulus that attempts to imitate the changing qualities of ongoing speech. They also include the hardware for an easy, fast measurement of RECD.

Once the client's own ear canal resonance or "ear print" is known, the RECD can be recorded and automatically factored into the equation for determining the DSL fitting targets. For the client, especially the child, this means that he or she no longer needs to be sitting in the room for subsequent probe tube (real ear) microphone measures. The clinician can simply connect the hearing to the 2-cc coupler, factor in the RECD, and predict with confidence that subsequent measures made this way will be very similar to any real ear measures that would be taken on the real client. All subsequent measures (e.g., with different hearing aid trimmer settings) can be made and the client technically no longer needs to be present. This facet of testing could be very useful when assessing the hearing aid function on the child with a short attention span who has "better" things to do.

Average RECD values can also be entered in the DSL computer fitting program, with these based on norms gathered from age groups that differ by each month up to the age of 5 years. Past the age of 5 years, there is no difference in the averaged RECD values, because the physical volume and size of the ear canal are assumed to plateau.

Unlike the other methods mentioned, DSL is concerned with "in situ" measures—not "insertion" measures. Insertion gain, for example, is commonly known as the difference between aided and unaided SPL at the eardrum. It does not consider or include the factors of head shadow, concha resonance, or ear canal resonance. In situ (in Latin it means "in situation," or "in place") gain, on the other hand, does not exclude these factors. The DSL method utilizes in situ measures because they include the factors that influence the output of the hearing aid on any particular person.

Another thing that sets DSL apart from its cousin fitting methods is that for DSL the output from the hearing aid is of final interest-not the gain. This has merit because it is the output, after all, that is the final delivered "goods" to the ear. In summary then, DSL looks at output that is derived from input and in situ gain measures.

The most unique facet of DSL is that all values on its fitting graph (SPL-o-gram) are in units of dB SPL, which enables everything to read in the "language" of hearing aid specifications (see Figure 3–6). The typical audiogram reads "downward" for increases in hearing loss, while increases in hearing aid gain and output on "spec" sheets are plotted in the opposite direction, can (and does) often lead to a lot of confusion. More confusion arises because intensity on typical audiograms is plotted in units of dB HL, while intensity on hearing aid specification sheets is plotted in dB SPL. The DSL fitting method circumvents these inconsistencies by plotting the audiogram "upside-down," with intensity in units of dB SPL. Low to high frequencies are plotted on the X axis from left to right, and intensity increases in dB SPL is plotted on the Y axis from the bottom upwards.

The normal human audibility curve is positioned at the bottom of the graph that shows the typical "smile" of poorer hearing sensitivity for the low and the very high frequencies (see Chapter 2). The "floor" of hearing loss is plotted higher up on the graph and can be readily visualized relative to normal hearing. The "ceiling" of loudness discomfort is positioned near the top of the graph. The unaided LTASS can also be seen as plotted across the frequencies of the graph. It now becomes readily apparent which speech sounds sit "below" the thresholds of the client and which speech sounds are audible. It can also be seen where the dynamic range for the client is largest and where it might become smaller. Of course, more compression will be needed for the narrow areas of the dynamic range.

The goal of DSL can readily be seen on the DSL graph and as mentioned earlier, this is to "raise" LTASS above the thresholds of the client

DSL "SPL-o-gram"

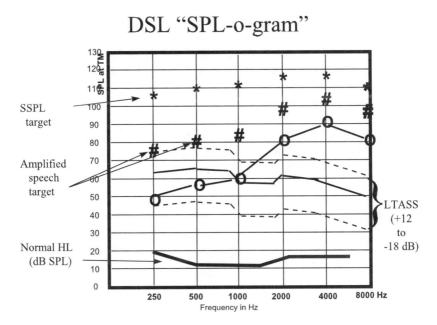

Figure 3–6. Unlike the typical audiogram, everything in DSL is plotted upwards in units of dB SPL. Normal hearing is shown as a curve, because it is now in SPL and the hearing loss goes up instead of down. Unaided speech or the long-term average speech spectrum (LTASS) has a 30 dB range. Mean SPL is shown by the solid line; the top dotted line is 12dB above the mean and the bottom dotted line is 18 dB below the mean. Speech is thus a sound that is not "normally" distributed around the mean. A target for amplification of average speech is situated in the person's dynamic range, between his or her hearing thresholds and SSPL targets. Note that all targets are plotted in terms of output—not gain. Note also that compression will be needed in the more narrow dynamic range at the high frequencies.

without exceeding his or her UCLs. As we have already seen in Figure 3-5, the high-frequency elements of speech have less intensity than the more tonal, low-frequency elements do. Furthermore, most people with SNHL have poorer hearing in the high frequencies. These two factors taken together with the stated DSL goal of making all of speech audible to the client, imply what has been stated earlier—namely, that DSL prescribes more high-frequency emphasis than most other hearing aid fitting methods.

The NAL-NL1 Fitting Method

As mentioned in Chapter 2, there is now a compression version of the NAL fitting method, the NAL-NL1, which stands for National Acoustics Laboratories, Non-Linear, version 1. This method appeared as of the very end of 1998, so it was not covered in the original printing of this little book. It just goes to show how fast things are evolving in the world of hearing aids and hearing aid fitting methods. The basic goals of the NAL-NL1 fitting methods are twofold: to maximize the intelligibility of speech and to restore normal loudness perceptions for speech. This last goal is similar to the restoration of loudness growth, the basic idea behind the IHAFF fitting method, as stated by Cox (1995), in which someone who wears hearing aids should perceive speech with the same loudness as someone who has normal hearing. In other words, the NAL-NL1 fitting method seeks to amplify the various frequency elements of speech so that they are at relative loudness levels that will most enhance the intelligibility of speech. Of course, the added corollary is that aided speech should sound just as loud as it would to those with normal hearing.

The NAL-NL1 fitting method, however, proposes that it differs from other suprathreshold fitting methods in that it does *not* try to preserve the normal loudness relationships among different frequency bands of speech. From looking at Figure 3-5, it can be seen that those who have normal hearing will hear the low-frequency elements of speech more loudly than the high-frequency elements of speech. While the other suprathreshold fitting methods might try to preserve this relationship, NAL-NL1, instead, adheres to the goals of NAL-R, in that it tries to make all frequency elements of speech be heard *equally loud.* The result would "flatten" the normally "sloped" relationship among the different frequencies of speech, so that the unvoiced consonants would no longer be quite as soft in comparison to the vowels. It may therefore be expected that NAL-NL1 will ask for less high-frequency gain or output than DSL. This is certainly the case when comparing the older, linear-based NAL-R to the POGO fitting method (see Chapter 2). Because the NAL-NL1 is such a new fitting method at this time, it is difficult to say just how it would compare to, for example, Fig6, IHAFF, or DSL.

The reason the NAL-NL1 fitting method deviates from the approach of preserving the unaided loudness relationships among the different frequency elements of speech is because the "preserving" approach has not been shown to improve speech intelligibility (Dillon, Katsch, Byrne, Ching, Keidser, & Brewer, 1998). Furthermore, according to Byrne, Parkinson, and Newall (1990), to achieve maximum intelligibility for speech, those with profound hearing loss require even less loudness for the high frequencies than those with other degrees of hearing loss. It is basically true that greater audibility implies greater loudness perception; but Dillon et al. (1990) found that, for profound hearing loss, the high frequencies contribute less to overall intelligibility of speech than they do for those with lesser degrees of hearing loss.

For the proponents of NAL-NL1, audibility is one thing, and *effective audibility* is another. Effective audibility is the *use* that those with hearing loss can make of audible speech, and for the designers of NAL-NL1, this decreases for increasing degrees of hearing loss, especially for those that exceed 40 dB HL. Someone with a profound hearing loss might be able to hear some particular element of speech, but may very well be completely unable to get any information from it. The NAL-NL1 fitting method assumes that effective audibility decreases with increased degree of hearing loss; that is, the use one can make of audible speech cues decreases as the hearing loss worsens. Furthermore, increased sensation levels or audibility of sound provide progressively less and less effective audibility as the hearing loss increases. For example, for perfectly effective audibility, someone with normal hearing may require a speech sound to be heard at a sensation level of about 40 dB, whereas someone with a severe-to-profound hearing loss may need the same speech sound to be just barely audible, or above his or her hearing threshold.

The NAL-NL1 fitting method basically differs from the DSL method in that it is especially concerned with "effective audibility," as well as with audibility of speech sounds. Accordingly, it can be assumed that NAL-NL1 will ask for less high-frequency gain (and output) than DSL. But it also differs in a few other ways. First, NAL-NL1 allows for the more traditional use of gain, as well as output. Second, the graphical displays mentioned in the NAL-NL1 user manual (version 1.01) include the audiogram in HL, 2-cc coupler gain, 2-cc coupler input-output curves, real ear insertion gain, real ear aided gain (i.e., in situ gain), a speech-o-gram, aided thresholds, among others. Third, the RECD, as asked for in DSL, is an added option, but it is not a central feature for NAL-NL1, because the targets can be indicated in terms of insertion gain (the difference between aided and unaided SPL at the eardrum). The NAL-NL1 user manual (version 1.01) suggests that, if the hearing aid is flexible in its trimmer settings, it can simply be inserted into the ear of the client and adjusted until the measured gain comes close to meeting the gain targets.

In conclusion, although NAL-NL1 has some very different assumptions and features, several DSL features are included in NAL-NL1. The speech-o-gram includes the 30 dB dynamic range of typical, long-term unaided speech, much like DSL. In addition, the aided thresholds can be read in terms of dB SPL or HL. In keeping with the knowledge that ear canal volumes and resonances for children are far different from those of adults, the user manual for NAL-NL1 duly notes an exception in measuring insertion gain for children; here, it is suggested that RECD be measured for the purpose of reducing probe microphone measures on squirming children, but also to allow for the fact that the ear canals in children are smaller and the resonances are higher than those for adults. Last, for children, the use of real ear aided gain (in situ gain) is suggested instead of insertion gain, because it takes into account these unique physical characteristics when predicting what the hearing aid will *actually* do when on the ear of the child. For DSL, imitation, it appears, is the finest form of flattery.

SUMMARY

■ Loudness growth, compression circuitry in hearing aids, and suprathreshold fitting methods all go together.
■ The thresholds of SNHL are worse than those of normal hearing, yet loudness tolerance is usually not much different from that of normal hearing. Instead of thinking of hearing loss thresholds as a below normal plot on an audiogram, it may help to flip the audiogram upside down, and think of them as the "floor" of hearing sensitivity being raised compared to that of normal hearing. Similarly, loudness tolerance can be seen as the "ceiling." In this way, we can consider the dynamic range being smaller than normal for hearing loss. A smaller dynamic range means a faster growth of loudness.
■ Compression circuitry, unlike linear circuitry, changes the gain depending on the input intensity level. Compression in general, gives a greater gain for soft input intensity levels, and less gain for more intense inputs. Soft input sounds below the "floor" of the hearing thresholds need to be amplified by a lot, while intense sounds that are near the "ceiling" do not need to be amplified by much at all. For those with smaller-than-normal dynamic ranges and consequently, faster-than-normal loudness growths, compression hearing aids may provide a better fit than linear hearing aids.
■ Suprathreshold fitting methods are based on restoring normal loudness growth with compression hearing aids. They all focus on speech as the target, which has its own unique properties, and they try to fit amplified speech into the smaller-than-normal dynamic range of the person with hearing loss.

RECOMMENDED READING

Mueller, G. H. (1997). 20 questions: Prescriptive fitting methods: The next generation. *The Hearing Journal, 50*(10), 10–19.
This reference cites several other sources. It also gives the phone numbers, faxes, and internet addresses for ordering any of the fitting methods described in this chapter.

CHAPTER 4

The Many Faces of Compression

Compression is *the* big word today in the realm of hearing aids. At almost every conference that has to do with hearing lately, there is some presentation that deals specifically with the issues of compression. Hearing aid specification sheets hail the advent and eminence of compression, and all kinds of compression hearing aids are sold by almost every hearing aid manufacturer.

Many clinicians readily admit they don't have a sound grasp on the many types of compression, nor do they readily know when to fit what type. Witness the way we scour the "specs" sheets on hearing aids, trying desperately to find those little words that will tell us once and for all what is what and when to fit what. Many graduate programs in audiology are guilty of not teaching compression very well, often because the professor of the hearing aids class does not really understand compression either. I should know. I taught a graduate course in hearing aids and did not have a good handle on the difference between input and output compression and when to fit what. I have since gained some understanding, but it is still a struggle to keep up with constantly changing jargon and terminology that hearing aid manufacturers use to tout their products.

In the preceding chapters the cochlea was presented as a magnificent nonlinear organ. Our attempts to restore "normal" hearing with imperfect technology and a myriad of fitting methods have not always been successful. We are taking small steps toward our goal, but they *are* in the right direction. This chapter covers compression hearing aids.

Compression has many faces. There is no one simple way to describe it cleanly. The best way to look at compression is like we do when we look at a sculpture. One needs to walk around it and see it from several different angles to appreciate it. This chapter aims at doing just that.

FIRST, A WORD ABOUT INPUT/OUTPUT GRAPHS

Input/output graphs are common to all specs sheets from any hearing aid manufacturer, so it may be a good idea to make them your friends. Ideally, clinicians should be able to ignore the written content on the specs sheets from any hearing aid manufacturer, look only at the graphs, and be able to tell what type of compression is being shown.

The graphs in Figures 4–1, 4–3 and 4–4 are input/output graphs, with the X axes showing input sound pressure level (SPLs) and the Y axes showing output SPLs. The lines on each graph are the "functions" and they represent the working of the hearing aid. The functions on each graph show the gain of a hearing aid for different input SPLs.

As discussed in Chapter 2, the most important formula for understanding hearing aid function is: input + gain = output. For each graph, "gain" is represented by the diagonal lines. The point where each gain line suddenly takes a bend is called the compression "threshold," or "kneepoint," and it is at this point that "compression" begins. The "kneepoint" of compression above the input axis shows the input SPL where compression begins. From now on, the term "kneepoint" is used to describe the input where compression begins.

The gain is linear to the left of the kneepoint, which means that for any increase of input SPL there is an equal increase of output SPL. For example, if the hearing aid has a gain of 50 dB, then a 10 dB SPL input will result in a 60 dB SPL output, a 20 dB SPL input results in a 70 dB SPL output, and so on. Linear gain was discussed in Chapter 2.

With compression, the gain is "nonlinear" because it *changes* as a function of input SPL. The slope of any line to the right of a compression kneepoint shows the effect of compression on the gain of the hearing aid. A compression kneepoint, for example, at an input of 70 dB SPL means that the hearing aid provides linear gain for input levels up to 70 dB SPL. For inputs above that intensity level, compression begins. When there is compression, an increase in input SPL does not result in an equal (linear) increase in output SPL. The gain for input SPLs "above" or to the right of the kneepoint is less than the gain for input SPLs "below" the kneepoint.

The maximum power output (MPO) is shown by the general "height" of any line that is to the right of the kneepoint. For input sound pressure levels to the right of the kneepoint, compression determines the MPO of the hearing aid.

Some hearing aids provide what is known as "curvilinear compression." This refers to the shape of the input-output line or function. Instead of having a sharp bend, the line takes a curve. The kneepoint is rounded instead of having a sharp corner. Curvilinear compression shows that the hearing aid gradually goes into its full degree or amount of compression; that is, the amount of compression increases gradually over increasing input levels.

INPUT COMPRESSION VERSUS OUTPUT COMPRESSION

Compression is often referred to as automatic gain control (AGC), because it changes the gain of the hearing aid as the input intensity SPL changes. In this chapter, the use of the word "compression" is used. When the clinician is confronted with compression, the first division that becomes apparent is the issue of input compression versus output compression. What is the difference and, furthermore, when does one fit which type?

When the author taught compression late in the semester's hearing aids class, he said that input compression hearing aids have a compressor located between the microphone and the amplifier and that output compression hearing aids have a compressor located between the amplifier and the receiver. Whether this is true or not is one thing; but it is of precious little value to the clinician fitting Mrs. McGillicudy who has presbycusis.

For the clinician, the big difference between input and output compression is where the *volume control* sits in the circuit (see bottom of Figure 4–1), because *it* is manipulated by the person who wears the hearing aid (at least on traditional hearing aid styles having user-controlled volume controls (VCs); this is changing with the introduction of more programmable and digital devices). If the VC has a different effect for input than it does for output compression, it behooves of the clinician to know what that difference is.

For output compression hearing aids, the VC is situated "early on" in the circuit; it is located between the microphone and the amplifier (Figure 4–1, bottom left). For input compression hearing aids, the VC is situated almost dead last in the circuit, just in front of the receiver that sends sound into the ear (Figure 4–1, bottom right).

Different VC locations lead to dramatic differences in what they do. The two graphs in Figure 4–1 show the different effects of the VCs with output compression hearing aids (top left) and input compression hearing aids (top right).

Input Versus Output Compression: Volume Control Effects

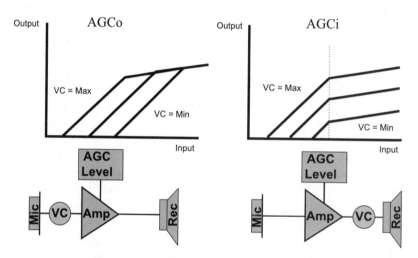

Figure 4–1. Input/output graphs and simple circuit schematics showing relative volume control positions for output compression (*left*) and input compression (*right*). For each graph, the parallel diagonal lines rising from the X axis represent linear gain; the corners represent the threshold kneepoint of compression; the line(s) to the right of the kneepoints represent the maximum power output (MPO). The position of the volume control in the circuits determines its effect. For output compression (*left*), the volume control affects gain and kneepoint, but not MPO. For input compression (*right*), the volume control affects gain and MPO, but not kneepoint.

Output Compression

For output compression hearing aids (Figure 4–1, top left), the VC affects the gain but not the MPO. The three diagonal gain lines in each graph show the effects of three different VC positions. The right-most line shows minimum gain, with the volume control position *lowered* to a minimum position. The left-most line shows maximum gain, with the volume control *raised* to a maximum position.

To make this clear, it may help to draw some more lines here. From the right-most kneepoint on the output compression graph, draw a vertical line down to the input axis. From the same kneepoint, draw a horizontal line to the output axis. This shows that at the minimum volume control setting, some X amount of input is needed to give some Y amount of output. If similar vertical and horizontal lines are drawn from the left-most kneepoint, it may become clear that for the maximum volume control position, less input is needed to give about the same amount of output. At low–volume positions, lots of input is needed to result in some amount of output. At high–volume positions, less input is needed to give about the same amount of output. This means that the gain is increased as the volume control position is raised.

The input/output graph also shows that once "past" or to the right of the kneepoint, in the region of compression, there is only one MPO line that is common to all three diagonal lines. This shows that, for output compression hearing aids, the volume control does not affect the MPO.

Note that the VC also changes the compression kneepoint. This is because the compression kneepoint is adjusted "later on" in the circuit after the volume control; the compressor is always set to wait for some steady amount of voltage that will tell it to compress (Figure 4-1, bottom left). The volume control affects the amount of input signal that will arrive at the compressor of the hearing aid. If this amount of input voltage is not enough to tell the compressor to compress, then it will not act. Only when the VC sends the required input signal voltage that the compressor is "waiting for," will the compressor then "do its thing."

Input Compression

For input compression hearing aids the effects of the VC are completely different (see Figure 4–1, top right). For input compression, the volume control affects both the gain *and* the MPO.

Again, three diagonal gain lines for three different volume control positions are shown. Again, the right-most diagonal gain line shows the lowest volume control setting, and the left-most gain line shows the highest or maximum volume control setting. It is obvious that the MPO is also affected by the volume control because once "past" or to the right of the kneepoint, the height of all three gain lines also changes.

Note also for input compression hearing aids, that the VC does not affect the kneepoint of compression. As Figure 4–1 (bottom right) shows, the compressor is situated before the VC. This means that the VC does nothing to the kneepoint because the compression kneepoint is already determined!

Input/output graphs are not the only way to look at the differences in the VC effects. The clinician is apt to be familiar with the frequency responses (gain as a function of frequency) seen on a hearing aid test box screen or printout, as shown in Figure 4–2. Here, the effects

Input Versus Output Compression: Volume Control Effects

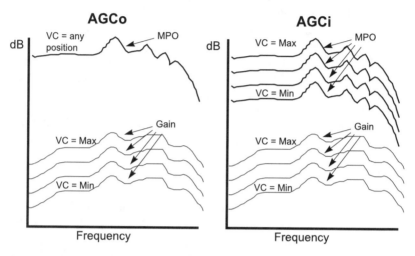

Figure 4–2. Frequency responses showing relative volume control positions for output compression (left) and input compression (right). Again, as shown in Figure 4–1, the volume control for output compression adjusts the gain, but not the MPO; for input compression, the volume control adjusts the gain along with the MPO.

of the VC on gain and MPO are readily apparent for output compression (left graph) in comparison to input compression (right graph). For output compression, the VC increases and decreases the gain; for input compression, both the gain and the MPO are affected by the VC.

Clinical Uses of Input and Output Compression

Input and output compression are not "better" or "worse" than each other; they are just different, and they have different clinical applications.

Output compression may be good for severe-to-profound hearing losses where the dynamic range is very small. For these clients, the clinician may worry that an excessively high VC position might cause damage to remaining hair cells or residual hearing; an output compression circuit will ensure that the VC affects only the gain and not the MPO. Output compression may also be good for children, for the same reason. The parent, teacher, or caregiver does not need to worry about excessive MPO when the little person runs into the house with the VC on a full-on position.

Input compression may be good for mild-to-moderate SNHL where the dynamic range is larger and there is consequently more room for "play" on MPO. As we have seen in Chapter 1, mild-to-moderate presbycusis is the most common type of hearing loss. Input compression hearing aids thus have a large potential fitting application.

COMPRESSION CONTROLS: CONVENTIONAL VERSUS "TK"

The issue of input and output compression can be left in the "rear view mirror" and we can turn now to another face of compression, the effect of manipulating another variable in hearing aids—namely, the compression kneepoint control. For this topic, think of the variable of VC as frozen in a constant position.

There are two types of compression kneepoint controls: (1) the earliest or original type, here called the conventional compression control, and (2) a compression control developed in the 1980s, commonly known as the threshold kneepoint (TK) control. The effect of each of these can be seen in Figure 4–3. Both graphs in the figure are once again, input/output graphs, similar to those in Figure 4–1.

Conventional Compression Control

The left graph in Figure 4–3 shows the effects of the conventional compression kneepoint control. It is typically found on output compression hearing aids, but also on some input compression hearing aids. At the present time, most input compression hearing aids have the TK control.

The conventional compression control affects the compression kneepoint and the MPO. It does so by adjusting the voltage level that the compressor of the circuit needs to begin compressing. As the control is turned to a maximum position, the compression kneepoint is raised, along with the MPO. At a maximum kneepoint setting, the compression hearing aid is in a linear gain mode for a wide range of soft to average input SPLs; compression will not occur until input sounds that are higher than the intensity level specified by the kneepoint are reached. At the maximum kneepoint setting, the MPO is also increased. Note from Figure 4–3 (left-most graph) that the conventional compression control does not affect the gain; the diagonal, linear gain line does *not* change with changes to the compression control settings.

The effects of this control can be heard in addition to being tested on a hearing aid test box; the cochlea is an excellent acoustic analyzer.

Different Ways of Adjusting AGC

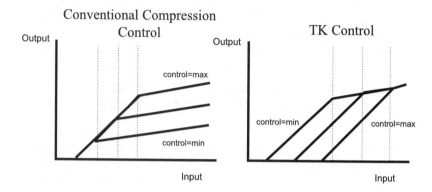

■ Compression Control: Affects Kneepoint & Output

■ "TK" Control: Affects Kneepoint & Gain

Figure 4–3. Input/output graphs showing effects of two different types of compression controls (volume control is assumed to be held constant at some position). For both graphs, the diagonal line(s) rising from the X axis represent linear gain; the corners represent the threshold kneepoint of compression; the line(s) to the right of the kneepoints represent the maximum power output (MPO). Both controls adjust the kneepoint of compression, but that is where the similarity ends. The conventional compression control affects MPO; the TK control affects gain for soft input pressure levels only.

To hear the effect of the typical compression control, you must speak *loudly* into the hearing aid, because only then will the input sound plus the gain reach the MPO (a low-intensity input sound, such as a soft voice, plus the gain of the hearing aid may not result in an output that reaches the MPO). As the compression control is turned from a maximum position to a minimum position, the kneepoint of compression and the MPO are reduced, you should notice that the amplified loud voice becomes softer. This is because the compression control affects the MPO, not the gain.

TK Control

The TK control is completely different. The right-most graph in Figure 4–3 shows the effect of the TK control. Technically, any compression control affects the kneepoint of compression, but electrical engineers will probably be quick to note that the term "threshold kneepoint" is an input-related term, and rarely encountered with output compression hearing aid circuitry. At any rate, the TK control is almost always found on input compression hearing aids. The term TK control is most often associated with K Amp™ hearing aids, and along with them, it has become known as a separate entity from regular compression controls.

The TK control affects the threshold kneepoint of compression and also the gain for soft input SPLs. This is because the TK control adjusts the kneepoint of compression over a range of relatively low input levels, from around 40 to 55 dB SPL. Like all compression hearing aids, those with the TK control provide greater, linear gain below the threshold kneepoint of compression. However, because this kneepoint is found at relatively soft inputs, the TK control can be seen as a gain booster for soft sounds. Unlike the conventional compression control, the TK control does not affect the MPO.

When listening to a hearing aid with a TK control, it is important to speak *softly* into the microphone to hear the effect of turning the control. With loud speech, the effect of the TK will seem minimal or not audible at all. This is very different from the conventional compression control where the sound becomes louder to the listener as the kneepoint is raised and the MPO is increased.

The input/output graph for the TK control (Figure 4–3, top right) looks similar to the graph showing the volume control effects for output compression (Figure 4–1, top left). This is because the TK control operates in a similar manner to the volume control for output compression hearing aids. The TK control is located at the input stage of the hearing aid (recall that the VC for output compression is positioned before the compressor and amplifier). It thus affects the amount of input signal that arrives at the compressor of the circuit, just like the VC does for output compression hearing aids.

Many clinicians have been confused by the TK control and how it works. It is very important to note that the left-most gain line, where there is greatest gain, shows the TK set to the *lowest* kneepoint position. The right-most gain line, where there is the least amount of gain, shows the TK set to the *highest* kneepoint position. As the compression kneepoint with the TK control is lowered, the gain for low-intensity input sounds is increased! Similarly, as the compression kneepoint with the TK control is raised, the gain for low-intensity input sounds is decreased.

Clinical Uses of Conventional and TK Compression Controls

Because the conventional compression control affects the MPO and not the gain, it can be used to *limit* the MPO to protect the client who wears the hearing aid from further hair cell damage and hearing loss. This type of compression control is especially useful for those clients who have a severe or profound hearing loss and a limited dynamic range. As mentioned earlier, this compression control is most often found on *output* compression hearing aids, which are also more suited for severe-to-profound hearing loss.

The purpose behind the TK control is an attempt to imitate the function of the outer hair cells (OHCs) of the cochlea (Killion, 1996). In Chapter 1, it was mentioned that the OHCs amplify soft sounds (approximately less than 40 to 50 dB SPL) so that the inner hair cells (IHCs) can sense them. Use of the TK control is therefore most appropriate for mild-to-moderate SNHL. As mentioned before, the TK control is most often associated with the kAmp™, which is a specific type of input compression hearing aid. This is discussed in further detail in the next section.

OUTPUT LIMITING COMPRESSION VERSUS WIDE DYNAMIC RANGE COMPRESSION (WDRC)

Two faces of compression have been discussed: (1) input versus output compression, and (2) the conventional compression control versus the TK control. A third face is "output limiting" compression versus "wide dynamic range" compression (WDRC). These are two different compression methods or philosophies-not specific controls. The effects of output limiting compression and WDRC can be seen in Figure 4–4. Once again, both graphs in the figure are input/output graphs, similar to those in Figure 4–1 and 4–3.

Output Limiting Compression

Output limiting compression is typically associated with *output* compression hearing aids that use a conventional compression control; but it can also be found on *some input* compression hearing aids, where compression is used for limiting the output.

The salient features of output limiting compression are shown in the left-most graph of Figure 4–4. Output limiting compression is as-

Compression Limiting Versus Wide Dynamic Range Compression

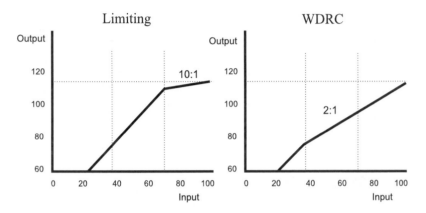

Figure 4–4. Input/output graphs showing effects of output limiting compression (left) and wide dynamic range compression (right). For both graphs, the diagonal lines rising from the X axis represent linear gain; the corners represent the threshold kneepoint of compression; the lines to the right of the kneepoint represent the MPO. In this example, the hearing aid gain is the same (60 dB) for each type of compression. The shape of the gain function, however, is very different for each type of compression. Output limiting compression has a high kneepoint and a high compression ratio; wide dynamic range compression has a low kneepoint and a low compression ratio.

sociated with *"high"* compression kneepoints and *high* compression ratios. A high kneepoint means that the hearing aid begins to compress at relatively high input SPLs (i.e., 55 to 60 dB SPL or more). Below the kneepoint, the hearing aid provides linear gain.

Compression ratios are the amount of compression provided by the hearing aid once compression begins. Compression ratios can be visualized on an input/output graph by the slant of the line after the kneepoint. A 10:1 compression ratio means that for every 10 dB increase of input SPL, there is only a 1 dB corresponding increase to the output SPL. A 2:1 compression ratio means that for every 10 dB increase of input SPL, there is a corresponding 5 dB increase to the output SPL of the hearing aid. A high compression ratio is usually defined as being greater than 5:1 (Dillon, 1988). Higher compression ratios, indicate *more* compression.

Output limiting compression hearing aids have a high kneepoint and a high ratio of compression. They provide a strong degree of compression over a narrow range of inputs (Figure 4–4, left graph). Below the threshold kneepoint, the output limiting compression hearing aid provides linear gain for a wide range of input SPLs. In other words, it "waits" for a fairly high input SPL to go into compression, but once it goes into compression, it *really* goes into compression.

Output limiting compression hearing aids have some similarities to linear hearing aids. They both give a fixed amount of gain over a wide range of different input SPLs, and then they both "suddenly" limit the output SPL. The main difference between them is that linear hearing aids use peak clipping to limit the output, and output limiting compression hearing aids use a high ratio of compression to limit the output. The advantage of limiting with compression is that it introduces less distortion than peak clipping.

Wide Dynamic Range Compression (WDRC)

WDRC hearing aids have become extremely popular during the past several years. It is important to categorize where WDRC properly fits in the overall spectrum of the many faces of compression, because then, it can be appreciated for what it is, and what it is not.

WDRC is shown in Figure 4–4 (right graph). The TK control is used to adjust WDRC and like the TK control, WDRC is almost always associated with *input* compression hearing aids. Recall, however, that not all input compression is WDRC; some input compression uses output limiting compression, which is adjusted by a conventional compression control.

WDRC is associated with *low* threshold kneepoints (below 55 dB SPL) and *low* compression ratios (less than 5:1). As the right-most graph of Figure 4–4 shows, the WDRC hearing aid is almost always in compression, because all kinds of inputs, from very soft speech to a scream, will cause it to go into compression. Perhaps it's called "wide dynamic range compression" because of its low kneepoint, which allows compression to take place over a wide range of input intensity levels.

Once the WDRC hearing aid goes into compression, however, it does not provide a great ratio or degree of compression (Figure 4–4). Basically, a WDRC hearing aid provides a weak degree of compression over a wide range of inputs. The effect of WDRC is very different from output limiting compression or linear hearing aids, for that matter. Unlike those hearing aids that suddenly reduce the gain once the input SPL exceeds a certain amount, WDRC gradually reduces the gain for a wide range of input SPLs.

Clinical Applications of Output Limiting Compression and WDRC

When comparing output limiting compression with WDRC, it may be most useful and helpful to look closely at their names. The main clinical difference between the two is that output limiting compression does its work *above* its kneepoint; it reduces or limits the output for high input SPLs. On the other hand, WDRC does its work *below* its kneepoint; it increases its gain for sounds below the kneepoint by providing most gain for soft input sounds (Johnson, 1993; Killion, 1996a).

Why would clinicians desire a choice between these two types of compression? To answer this question, it may be a good idea to take another look at loudness growth, already discussed in Chapter 3. The client who has OHC damage usually has a mild-to-moderate SNHL. For this person, the "floor" of hearing sensitivity is elevated compared to normal, although the "ceiling" of loudness tolerance is similar to normal. The appropriate goal of amplification is to restore normal loudness growth and to accomplish this goal, we need to amplify soft sounds by a lot, and loud sounds by little or nothing at all.

Here is some food for thought: It is no coincidence that, on the one hand, the KAmpTM, WDRC, and on the other, otoacoustic emissions and the knowledge of the role of the OHCs, became clinically popular at around the same time-the late 1980s and early 1990s.

Figure 4–5 shows output limiting compression (left) and WDRC (right) superimposed on two identical loudness growth graphs. Both graphs are the same as that of Figure 3–1, which shows the loudness growth functions of someone with normal hearing compared to that of someone with a mild-to-moderate SNHL.

Figure 4–5 shows that both output limiting compression and WDRC may do the same thing for inputs of 90 dB; they may both reach the point where output sounds are perceived as being "too loud," but the *way* that each type of compression arrives at this common point is completely different. The author once attended an American Academy of Audiology conference seminar on compression given by F. Kuk in 1996, who provided a very illustrative analogy. Output limiting compression was compared to a teenager speeding down the road in a relative's car who sees a stop sign at the end of the road and slams on the brakes and screeches to a stop. WDRC was compared to an elderly person who starts out at a normal speed, but on seeing the stop sign far ahead, ever-so cautiously applies a foot gently to the brakes and slows to a stop over a long distance.

In the above analogy, normal loudness growth is the road. Some problems occur when trying to restore normal loudness growth with out-

Loudness Growth
&
Types of Compression

Output Limiting   WDRC

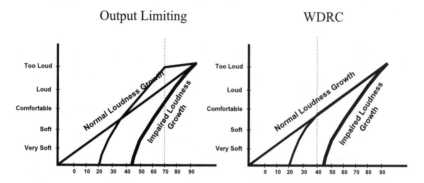

Figure 4–5. Re-establishing normal loudness growth with output limiting compression and wide dynamic range compression (WDRC). The X axis represents the physical dimension of input sound intensity to the hearing aid; the Y axis represents the psychoacoustic dimension of loudness perception (similar to Figure 3–1). In this example, both output limiting compression and wide dynamic range compression make 90 dB inputs sound "too loud." But the high kneepoint and high compression ratio for output limiting compression make inputs of 70, 80, and 90 dB all sound "too loud." This does not occur for WDRC, because it has a low kneepoint and a low compression ratio.

put limiting compression (Figure 4–5 left-most graph). First, there is an "overshoot" of normal loudness growth. The worst problem, however, is that amplified 70, 80, and 90 dB inputs all sound the same and are perceived as being "too loud." This does not restore normal loudness growth. The right-most graph shows WDRC applied to the same goal of restoring normal loudness growth. If restoring loudness growth is the goal, then the lower kneepoint and lower compression ratio that are provided by WDRC are clearly a much better fit, because soft sounds are perceived as louder, while loud sounds do not exceed the listener's comfort levels.

Maybe another reason for the term "WDRC" is that the low kneepoint and low compression ratio reduce a normally large dynamic range into the smaller one associated with mild-to-moderate SNHL. For example, a low compression ratio of 2:1 will compress a dynamic range of 100 dB into one of 50 dB.

Does this mean that we should all drive like the elderly person? Not really. A client with mild-to-moderate hearing loss may be used to wearing linear hearing aids. For this client, a sudden switch to WDRC might be too big a jump, and WDRC might be rejected because it is not "loud" enough. Although WDRC will amplify soft input SPLs by a lot, it will not amplify average intensity input SPLs by the same amount, and it is *this* that the client accustomed to linear amplification may find frustrating. Output limiting compression may result in the "overshoot" of normal loudness growth as seen in the left graph of Figure 4–5, but the client may have become accustomed to the sound. In this case, WDRC must be introduced gradually and with considerable counseling about what to expect from the hearing aids. Many such clients can adjust to WDRC, but others cannot seem to let go of their need for more power and refuse to make the change.

For the client with severe-to-profound hearing loss, output limiting compression might be a better choice than WDRC. These clients might prefer a strong, linear gain over a wide range of input SPLs, at least until the output SPL becomes close to their loudness tolerance or uncomfortable loudness levels. Furthermore, these clients often have worn powerful linear hearing aids in the past. Output limiting compression hearing aids, like their old linear hearing aids, will give lots of gain for soft sounds and the same "lots of gain" for average input sounds. Output limiting compression hearing aids have similar gain characteristics as linear hearing aids, and the client may appreciate these (see Chapter 6).

Hearing aids with output limiting compression still have a big advantage over linear hearing aids; for intense input SPLs, output limiting compression does not give the degree of distortion that is associated with the peak clipping of linear hearing aids. They may definitely be preferred by clients with severe-to-profound hearing loss.

BILL, TILL, AND MULTICHANNEL HEARING AIDS

It is hard to miss the relatively recent hype about multichannel hearing aids with WDRC. These are rapidly becoming *the* high-end hearing aids that promise maximum fitting flexibility, normal loudness growth for many different hearing loss configurations, and a natural and high quality of sound. Many manufacturers now have their own version of these types of hearing aids. These need not be listed here; the reader can simply glance at the vast amount of literature that is provided by the manufacturers and will be rewarded by a bombardment of information.

A Canadian company, the Gennum Corporation of Burlington Ontario, has produced a two-channel WDRC circuit known as the DynamEQII™. This circuit has been used by many manufacturers of hearing aids to create their own two-channel WDRC hearing aids. Some other manufacturers, such as ReSound, have their own proprietary multichannel circuits that provide WDRC.

BILL and TILL: Two Types of WDRC

Bass increase at low levels (BILL) and treble increases at low levels (TILL) are two types of WDRC. There are other names that pertain to these categories, such as LDFR (level-dependent frequency response), FDC (frequency-dependent compression), and ASP (automatic signal processing). Basically, these terms all boil down to at least one similar thing; namely, compression occurs more in some frequencies than in other frequencies. Where compression occurs the most, it will be WDRC, with a low kneepoint and a low compression ratio. The simplest classification of these types of compression is that of BILL and TILL (Killion, Staab, & Preves, 1990).

To understand BILL and TILL, it is first important to know that in any compression hearing aid, the compression kneepoint occurs at a different input SPL for different frequencies. BILL and TILL, however, are hearing aids where the kneepoint compression occurs at *very* different input SPLs for different frequencies.

That compression may occur more at some frequencies than at others, is not evident from the input/output graphs on hearing aid specs sheets. When hearing aid specs sheets in North America show the compression kneepoint, they adhere to the standards of the American National Standards Institute (ANSI, S3.22). This set of standards shows the compression kneepoint on these graphs as we have seen in Figures 4–1, 4–3, and 4–4, and input/output graphs do not show frequency. The ANSI standard specifies that the kneepoint of compression is to be shown on input/output graphs at one frequency, 2000 Hertz (Hz).

BILL hearing aids have a low kneepoint for the low frequencies and a higher kneepoint for the high frequencies. Low-frequency input will not have to be very intense to set the BILL hearing aid into compression. This means that the BILL circuit will go into compression very often with low-frequency inputs, and not as often with high-frequency inputs.

Figure 4–6 shows a simple set of gain and frequency graphs for BILL (left graph) and TILL (right graph) circuits. The BILL hearing aid (left graph) has a very broad or flat frequency response with soft in-

BILL Versus TILL

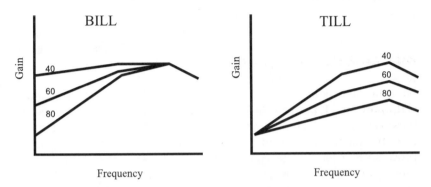

Figure 4–6. For each graph, the gain (Y axis) across a frequency range (X axis) is shown for three different input levels. The left graph shows bass increases at low levels (BILL). As inputs decrease in intensity, low-frequency gain increases. Examples of BILL are the Manhattan circuit ™ and the Oticon Multifocus™. The right graph shows treble increase at low levels (TILL). As inputs decrease in intensity, high-frequency gain increases. The KAmp™ is an example of a TILL circuit.

puts (e.g., 40 dB SPL). If input sound is produced so that it is at 40 dB SPL all across the frequency range, then the gain and frequency response of the BILL hearing aid will look something like the top flat line on the graph. As the input across frequencies is increased in intensity, to 60 dB SPL, the gain and frequency response will reveal a decrease in gain for the low frequencies. As the input intensity is increased to 80 dB SPL, the gain for the low frequencies will drop even more.

The main idea behind the BILL circuit is to enable better listening for speech while in background noise. That is, the "hubbub" of low-frequency background noise will be suppressed by compression, with the high-frequency sounds that render clarity for speech still receiving a full measure of gain. BILL was originally associated with the Argosy Manhattan circuit™. The hearing aid most commonly thought of when BILL is brought up today is the Oticon Multifocus™.

The TILL hearing aid (right graph) is completely different. The kneepoint is set at a low kneepoint for the high frequencies. For the TILL hearing aid, high-frequency input will not have to be very intense to cause compression. This means the TILL circuit will go into compression very often with high-frequency inputs, and not as often with low-frequency inputs.

Figure 4–6 (right graph) shows a TILL response. For the TILL hearing aid, low-intensity input SPLs of 40 dB across the frequency range will result in a gain and frequency response that has more of a high-frequency emphasis. As the input is increased to 60 dB SPL, the high-frequency emphasis will decrease relative to the gain for the low frequencies. With inputs of 80 dB SPL, the gain for the high frequencies will decrease even more. In some TILL in-the-ear hearing aids, the 80 plus dB SPL response is intended to resemble the resonance of the open, unaided ear, thus providing an acoustic "transparency" for intense inputs when amplification is not needed.

The main idea behind TILL is to emphasize the high-frequency sounds of speech for the listener who most typically has high-frequency hearing loss. As discussed in Chapter 3, this client will have a reduced dynamic range for the high frequencies. Compared to that for normal hearing, the "floor" of hearing sensitivity will be elevated, although the "ceiling" of loudness tolerance will not be. The hearing aid most commonly thought of when TILL is brought up today is the K Amp™.

Multichannel Hearing Aids

Today, both BILL and TILL are commonly combined into one hearing aid that has two or more channels (Figure 4–7). A multichannel hearing aid is like having two or more hearing aids in one. The term multichannel should not be confused with programmable; these two terms are mutually exclusive and they are very different things. Multichannel hearing aids *can* be programmable, but so can single-channel hearing aids. More will be discussed about programmable hearing aids in Chapter 5. For now, multichannel hearing aids are discussed without relationship to programmability. Because most multichannel hearing aids have two channels, the following discussion pertains to the popular Gennum DynamEQII™ two-channel hearing aid, with WDRC in each channel.

This two-channel circuit uses input compression, which can be determined from the position of the VC in the circuit (see Figure 4–7, right side). Figure 4–7 shows there is one microphone, followed by a band splitter, which separates the incoming input sound into two frequency bands, or channels. Each separate channel has its own amplifier and compressor.

The same circuit is also WDRC, with a single TK control to adjust the kneepoint of compression for both channels together. Figure 4–7 shows that the DynamEQII™ circuit combines BILL and TILL into one hearing aid. A BILL response is obtained if the gain of the low-frequency channel is turned up while that of the high-frequency channel is turned down. This could be a good setting for a "reverse" hearing

Multichannel Amplification
with
BILL & TILL

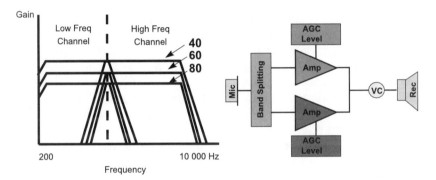

Figure 4–7. A two-channel WDRC hearing aid can be set up to produce a response of BILL, TILL, or both. On the right, a schematic for a two-channel compression hearing aid is shown. Following the microphone, a band splitter separates the inputs into a low-frequency band and a high-frequency band. Each frequency band is separately amplified and compressed. The end result is reunited into one receiver. There is also only one volume control. The gain and frequency graph on the left shows a two-channel WDRC hearing aid that is set up for both BILL and TILL. In this example, the client may have a "flat" hearing loss configuration. The two-channel WDRC hearing aid can also be set up to accommodate high- or low-frequency hearing losses.

loss configuration. A TILL response is obtained if the gain of the low channel is turned down while that of the high channel is turned up. This could be a good setting for a high-frequency hearing loss. Lastly, if the gain of both channels is turned up the same, then the circuit provides a BILL and a TILL response together, which could be a good setting for a "flat" hearing loss.

An especially interesting feature of the DynamEQII™ circuit is that the gain controls for each channel actually adjust the *compression ratio* for each channel. In most hearing aids that use this circuit, therefore, the threshold kneepoint can be adjusted for both channels together, while the compression ratios can be adjusted separately for each channel. An example of a two-channel hearing aid developed from the DynamEQII™ circuit is the Sound FX™ by Unitron Industries Ltd. More is discussed about the trimmers and the fitting rationale of this flexible hearing aid in Chapter 6. Some case studies of actual fittings with this multichannel WDRC hearing aid are also described in Chapter 6.

DYNAMIC ASPECTS OF COMPRESSION

Until now, compression has been discussed in terms of threshold knee-point and compression ratio. These are sometimes known as the "static" aspects of compression, because they involve the input SPL when compression begins and the degree of compression once it occurs. Sound in the environment, however, is constantly changing in intensity over time and a compression hearing aid has to respond to these changes in intensity over time. The "dynamic" aspects of compression are known as the "attack" and the "release" times.

The attack and release times are the lengths of time it takes for a compression circuit to respond to changes in the intensity of an input SPL (see Figure 4–8). When the input SPL exceeds the kneepoint of compression, the hearing aid "attacks" the sound by reducing the gain. Once the input sound falls below the kneepoint of compression, the hearing aid "releases" from compression and restores the gain. The attack time is the length of time it takes for a hearing aid to go into compression and reduce the gain; the release time is the length of time it takes for it to come out of compression and restore the gain.

An electrical circuit cannot instantly mirror the changes that take place in the environment, because it requires time to respond to these changes (Dillon, 1988). For example, if a compression circuit is to respond to a sudden input SPL increase, it has to wait for at least one cycle of the sound wave to "know" if the increased SPL will remain. A change in gain that occurs faster than the longest cycle or period of incoming sound can change the fine details of the sound waves and distortion will result.

Hearing aids are not the only electrical devices that use compression and have attack/release times. Audiovisual equipment has used input and output compression for many years and we have heard its effects before. Recall, for example, the television broadcasts in which the sports announcer is talking and the background noise is changing in intensity over time. When a score is made and the audience suddenly increases their cheers, the background noise increases in intensity. It may take a short time for the compression of the audiovisual equipment to attack and reduce the gain of the noise; but this also temporarily reduces the gain for the announcer's voice. When the cheering stops, it may again take some time for the system to release from

Dynamic Characteristics of Compression

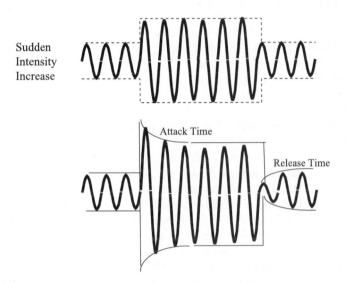

Sudden
Intensity
Increase

Attack Time

Release Time

Figure 4–8. The top shows a simple description of input sound changing in intensity (vertical dimension) over time (horizontal dimension). The sound has suddenly increased in intensity and after a while the sound suddenly decreases in intensity. The bottom shows the *output* response of a compression hearing aid to the changes in sound input intensity over time. The compression circuitry takes some amount of time to respond or compress the incoming signal that has suddenly increased in intensity. This is the "attack" time. Once the input sound has decreased in intensity, the circuit takes some time to stop compressing. This is the "release" time.

compression; and the announcer's voice will accordingly take some time to return back to a normal, audible level.

Most attack and release times are set to achieve a best compromise between two undesirable extremes. Times that are too fast will cause the gain to fluctuate rapidly and this may cause a jarring, "pumping" perception by the listener. Times that are too slow may make the compression act too slowly and cause a real lagging perception on the part of the listener. Quick attack times (i.e., 10 ms or less) might prevent sudden, transient sounds from becoming too loud for the listener. In general, release times need to be longer than attack times to prevent a "fluttering" perception on the part of the listener (Staab, 1996). Longer release times (i.e., up to 150 ms) tend to prevent severe distortions that occur with fast release times. Inordinately fast release times can cause the hearing aid to track the amplitude of individual cycles of sound waves (Staab, 1996). Such a rapid modulation of sound can cause a "breathing" or "pumping" perception on the part of the listener (Armstrong, 1996).

Just as we have seen with the static aspects of compression, there are lots of "buzz" words that float around when the dynamic aspects of compression are discussed. Different attack and release times are sometimes used to categorize different types of dynamic compression. Various types of dynamic compression methods are discussed briefly below.

Automatic Volume Control (AVC)

A type of compression known as "automatic volume control" (AVC) has often been used during broadcasts with audiovisual equipment. During televised sports events, AVC contributes to the time lag or delay in loudness changes in the announcer's voice, relative to the sudden-onset cheers of the audience. AVC has a relatively long attack and long release times; its release times are usually more than 150 ms and can be as long as several seconds (Hickson, 1994). Because of this, it does not respond to rapid fluctuations of sound input. On the contrary, it responds mainly to general, overall changes in sound intensity, which reduces the need for the listener to adjust the volume control manually: hence, its name.

Syllabic Compression

"Syllabic compression" is known for its relatively short attack and release times; its release times vary from less than 50 ms up to 150 ms. The attack/release times are specifically intended to be shorter than the duration of the typical speech syllable, which is about 200 to 300 ms (Hickson, 1994). Short attack/release times allow the hearing aid to compress or reduce the gain for the peaks of more intense speech (usually the vowel sounds), and this provides more uniformity in the intensity of ongoing speech syllables. In other words, syllabic compression reduces the differences between the normally more intense vowels and the softer unvoiced consonants such as /s/. The main premise of syllabic compression is to allow a hearing aid to make the softer sounds of speech more audible without simultaneously making the normally louder parts of speech from becoming too loud.

Syllabic compression is somewhat controversial and not everyone agrees with its use. Because syllabic compression compresses the peaks of speech and makes the waveform of ongoing speech more uniform, noise can easily fill in the small gaps that remain (Johnson, 1993), and in noisy situations, a hearing aid might amplify the noise that is situated between the peaks of speech. According to Killion (1996a), fast attack/release times of 50 ms can distort the waveform of speech, and, thus, compromise speech intelligibility.

Peak Detection

Most compression hearing aids have used a technique called peak detection to "track" the peak amplitude of incoming sound waves. If the peak is greater than the compression threshold kneepoint, the circuit attacks and begins to compress the signal, which reduces the gain. Once the peak is below the kneepoint, the compression releases and the gain increases again. Peak detection allows for a wide variety of times that can separately be specified and assigned as attack and release times; however, these times are constant and fixed for any incoming sound intensity patterns (Armstrong, 1993). Most peak detection systems in hearing aids are adjusted to provide *quick* attack times and *longer, slower* release times.

An advantage of peak detection is that it reacts very quickly to increases in environmental sound levels. Unfortunately, however, it can react inappropriately to very short intense sounds, because the longer release times will keep the gain down after the short intense sound has stopped. This may unnecessarily reduce the gain of sounds the listener might want to hear.

With fixed attack/release times, the hearing aid cannot respond differently to different patterns of sound input intensities when needed. As discussed in Chapter 2, speech is an example of sound that is constantly changing over time. The dynamic acoustic sounds of speech within the world of ever-changing background noise (e.g., the sudden slamming of a door or the constant roar of traffic) can pose real problems for the peak detection method and the listener.

Adaptive Compression™

This type of compression has fixed, quick attack times, but has release times that vary with the length or duration of the intense, incoming sound. For sudden intense transient sound inputs, the release time is short and for sound inputs that are longer in duration, the release times are longer. The desired result is a reduction of compression "pumping" heard by the listener. Adaptive compression™ was originally patented by Telex and it is most commonly associated with the K Amp™ circuits.

Average Detection

Average detection is most commonly associated with the DynamEQII™ circuit by Gennum (see the previous section on multichannel hearing aids). Unlike the peak detection method that tracks the peak amplitude of incoming sound waves, the average detection method looks at the average of incoming signal over a given length of time. When the average SPL exceeds the kneepoint of compression, then the gain is reduced.

The DynamEQII™ has "twin" average compression detectors; one is a fast detector and the other is a slow detector (see Figure 4–9). The slow average detector averages sound inputs over a 220 ms time interval (i.e., about 1/5 of a second) and it is in control of the compression system most of the time. When the slow average of incoming

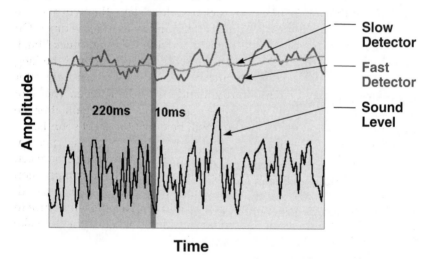

Twin Average Compression Detectors
for the DynamEQ™ Circuit

Figure 4–9. The figure shows the actions of the slow average detector, which averages sound over time intervals of about 220 ms, and the fast average detector, which averages sound over time intervals of about 10 ms. The bottom line represents sound intensity as it occurs over time. The top smooth line represents the input signal when averaged by the slow average detector. Note that the slow average is very flat over time. The top bumpy line represents the input signal when averaged by the fast detector. Note the fast average changes a lot more over time than the slow average, and it is thus more sensitive to sudden changes in sound intensity.

sounds exceeds the threshold kneepoint of compression, the gain is slowly reduced and is hardly noticeable. Very often, however, sudden loud sounds occur in the environment, and the gain needs to be reduced for these as well. For example, with the slow detector alone, a short spike of intense sound may be averaged into the overall body of sound that takes place over 220 ms. This slow average may not be enough to "tell" the hearing aid to go into compression and reduce the gain. This is where the fast average detector comes into the picture. The fast average detector averages sound inputs over time intervals of about 10 ms (i.e., 1/100 of a second) and it acts when intense transients are not "caught" by the slow detector. When the "fast" average is 6dB greater than the "slow" average, the fast average detector takes over and reduces the gain for the spike of intense sound.

The main result of twin average detection is that both the attack and release times vary with the length of the incoming intense sounds. This is in direct contrast to the peak detection systems that give constant, fixed quick attack and slow release times for all incoming stimuli. As long as the incoming sounds are below the compression threshold, both types of circuits provide uncompressed gain. With sudden transient loud sounds, however, such as a door slam, the twin average detection system will provide quick attack and quick release times. On the other hand, the peak detector will provide its usual quick attack and slow release times. Because of the reduction of gain and the long recovery of the peak detection circuit, soft speech spoken right after the door slam may be temporarily inaudible to the listener. The twin average detection circuit will enable a quick recovery of gain after the door slam, because, its release time will be quick for short sounds.

The benefit to the listener is that there is less "pumping" perception. The twin average detection system is a compromise between compression that reacts to every short intense sound and compression that may react too slowly for some sounds that should be compressed. Audible by-products of compression should not become a nuisance to listeners. Dynamic aspects should be considered when trying to make hearing aids acoustically "transparent."

INTERACTION BETWEEN STATIC AND DYNAMIC ASPECTS OF COMPRESSION

Compression consists of static aspects in one dimension and dynamic aspects in a purely separate dimension. With incoming sounds, the attack/release times of a hearing aid interact with the ratio of compression

(Armstrong, 1996). The input/output graphs on hearing aid spec sheets show compression ratios that are obtained with constant pure tones, not the stops and starts of sounds like speech. Static compression ratios on specs sheets do not accurately represent the actual compression ratios experienced in real life by clients who wear the hearing aids. Fast attack/release times have the effect of temporarily *reducing* the ratio or amount of compression for any given sound stimulus.

Attack and release times interact with compression ratios and these interactions affect the sound quality for the listener. In general, a combination of short attack/release times (e.g., 10 ms) and high compression ratios (e.g., 10:1) cause distortion. If the same short attack/release times are used with low compression ratios (e.g., 2:1), then the sound quality is not as distorted (Armstrong, 1996). On the other hand, long attack/release times can be combined with either high or low compression ratios.

Dynamic aspects and static aspects of compression are often found in predictable combinations today. Syllabic compression, with its relatively short attack and release times is most often associated with WDRC hearing aids that have a low-compression kneepoint and a low-compression ratio of less than 5:1. It is less common with output limiting compression hearing aids where the kneepoints and ratios of compression are "high." AVC, with its relatively long attack/release times, is most often seen in hearing aids that offer a low-threshold kneepoint of compression and high-compression ratio (Dillon, 1988; Hickson, 1994).

SUMMARY

- In this chapter, we have looked at some of the many faces of compression. With input/output graphs, compression was explored along three angles or dimensions: (X) input versus output compression, (Y) the conventional compression control versus the "TK" control, and (Z) output limiting compression versus WDRC.
- From a clinician's point of view, the main difference between input and output compression is the effect of the volume control. With output compression, the volume control affects the gain but not the MPO. With input compression, the volume control affects both the gain and the MPO.

- The effects of the conventional compression control and the TK control were compared, with the VC held constant. The conventional compression control affects the threshold kneepoint of compression and also the MPO. The TK control affects the kneepoint and the gain for soft inputs only. The effect of the conventional compression control is audible only when speaking loudly into the hearing aid; the effect of the TK control is audible only when speaking softly into the hearing aid.

- Output limiting compression was compared to WDRC regarding compression kneepoints and compression ratios. Output limiting compression has a high kneepoint, which means that compression is activated only for relatively intense sound input levels; it also has a high compression ratio. WDRC has a low kneepoint and a low compression ratio. These differences separate their respective clinical purposes. Output limiting acts mostly above its kneepoint to limit the output. WDRC acts mostly below its kneepoint to provide most gain for soft input sounds.

- Output compression is most often associated with output limiting compression and it is adjusted by a conventional compression control. It can be very appropriate for severe-to-profound hearing loss that usually exhibits a narrow dynamic range. Input compression is often associated with WDRC, and it is adjusted with a TK control. It can be very appropriate for mild-to-moderate SNHL, which usually exhibits a wider dynamic range.

- Mild-to-moderate SNHL is very common and WDRC is also becoming very popular. Two types of WDRC are BILL and TILL. Multichannel hearing aids that can combine BILL and TILL into one hearing aid are more flexible than single-channel WDRC hearing aids. These multichannel hearing aids are becoming very popular. The DynamEQII™ is an example of a two-channel WDRC circuit that can provide either BILL, TILL, or both.

- Dynamic aspects of compression were discussed separately from the static compression aspects of compression threshold knee point and compression ratio. Different types of attack/release time parameters were discussed. The usual compromise has been to provide fast attack times with longer release times. The newer twin average detection system has variable attack and release times. It is available on the new two-channel WDRC circuit called the DynamEQ™ circuit. This circuit is available through many hearing aid manufacturers.

RECOMMENDED READING

Dillon, H. (1988). Compression in hearing aids. In R. E. Sandlin (Ed.), *Handbook for hearing aid amplification* (Vol. I). Boston: College Hill.

Compression handbook: An overview of the characteristics and applications of compression amplification. 1996 Eden Prairie, MN: Starkey Marketing Services, Starkey Labs, Inc., 1996.

CHAPTER 5

Programmable and Digital Hearing Aids

In the last chapter we discussed the many types of compression, covering many of the "buzzwords" often encountered in the literature and in hearing aid specification sheets. A discussion of compression, however, would be incomplete without some discussion on programmable and digital hearing aids and how compression can be utilized in these types of circuits.

Programmable and digital hearing aids have become quite popular today. Almost every hearing aid manufacturer has at least one programmable hearing aid, and digital hearing aids are being developed and released by various manufacturers just about as fast as this book is being written. The pace of hearing aid technology development has quickened, and there is healthy competition among the manufacturers. This chapter presents the general aspects of programmable and digital hearing aids. A competitive comparison and contrast of these types of hearing aids is not covered in this chapter; instead, the respective advantages of programmable and digital hearing aids are discussed. One example of an analog, programmable hearing aid and two examples of the earliest fully digital hearing aids also are provided.

First, the terms "programmable" and "digital" should not be confused. Many hearing aids are "digitally programmable," but this does not necessarily mean that the circuit of the hearing itself provides digital signal processing (DSP). Many analog (i.e., not DSP) hearing aids are digitally programmable, but this simply means that instead of requiring that the clinician employ a screwdriver, the hearing aid trimmer settings and/or VC can be programmed by a hand-held programmer or by a computer with software created by some specific manufacturer. The only thing that is digital about analog programmable hearing aids is the computer used to program them. Computers are digital in that they use a complex series of binary mathematical sequences (i.e., a series of 0's and 1's. The Gennum DynamEQ™ circuit, used by many manufacturers to build their multichannel WDRC hearing aids, is an analog circuit; it is also available in a programmable version by some manufacturers.

ANALOG PROGRAMMABLE HEARING AIDS

In this section, the term "programmable" is used for analog (nondigital) hearing aids; digital, or DSP, hearing aids are described later as a completely separate entity. Although the DSP hearing aids available today can be programmed, it may be easier to understand the terms "programmable" and "digital" when described separately.

In the early 1990s, analog (nondigital), programmable hearing aids began to appear. Many of these were single-channel hearing aids where the clinician adjusted and set (i.e., programmed) the hearing aid trimmers with a computer or a hand-held programming unit. Programmable hearing aids can provide essentially the same compression characteristics as nonprogrammable hearing aids; the only difference is in the way that the controls or trimmers are accessed (programmability implies that no manual screwdriver manipulation is required).

Many programmable hearing aids offer two or more memories (i.e., programs); these provide clients access to different frequency responses with the flick of a switch, located on either the actual hearing aids, or on a hand-held remote-control device. By accessing different frequency responses, clients can personally adjust the hearing aids for optimal listening in different listening environments.

Programmable Hearing Aids Versus Multichannel Hearing Aids

At this point, it is important to discuss how programmable and multichannel hearing aids are totally separate concepts; once this is understood, it is less confusing to understand how they can intersect or be combined. Programmable hearing aids can be single-channel or multichannel (multichannel hearing aids were discussed in Chapter 4). However, a programmable hearing aid is not necessarily multichannel, nor is a multichannel hearing necessarily programmable. These properties can be combined, however, and any look at the offerings by manufacturers will quickly verify that combinations of programmable, multichannel hearing aids abound.

Some programmable hearing aids are single-channel. Single-channel, programmable hearing aids may have circuitry similar to nonprogrammable, single-channel hearing aids; the only difference between programmable, single-channel hearing aids and their nonprogrammable counterparts is that the clinician can set or adjust the trimmers by a computer or hand-held programmer. In Chapter 4, it was mentioned that in multichannel hearing aids, a band splitter divides the input sound into two or more bands, with each band having its own amplifier and perhaps, compressor. In a single-channel, programmable hearing aid, the incoming sound input is not split into two or more parts.

Single-channel programmable hearing aids often have programmable trimmer settings and, in some of these hearing aids, the VC may be also be programmable. Some examples of programmable trimmer settings include: MPO, gain, low-cut, high-cut, compression threshold kneepoint, ratio of compression, and attack/release times. The software provided by various manufacturers might suggest some practical trimmer settings that tend to work well with each other, depending on the degree and slope of someone's hearing loss. As mentioned earlier, the VC can also be programmed to be set at any particular position.

Single-channel programmable hearing aids can have one or more memories, or programs. Figure 5–1 shows a single-channel programmable circuit with two programs (left), compared to a multichannel circuit described earlier (right). Multichannel hearing aids can also be programmable: but most of these have only one program or memory. In other words, most multichannel programmable hearing aids can be programmed, but the end user cannot voluntarily toggle between alternate programs of the hearing aids. With the exception of an analog, multichannel, multiprogram hearing aid manufactured and patented by 3M (ReSound), other analog, multichannel hearing aids usually have one program.

A programmable hearing aid with two or more memories or programs enables the listener to manually adjust (by a switch on the hearing aid or by remote control) among the different programs. Figure 5–2 shows an example of a two-program, single-channel hearing aid that is set to meet the needs of someone who wants the ability to choose between two different sound programs: one program that will provide optimal gain for listening in quiet or for listening to music, and so on, where the widest frequency response may be desired, and the other

Programmable Versus Multichannel

Programmable

Multichannel

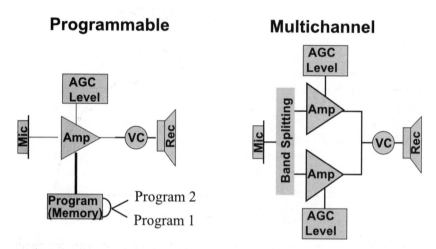

Figure 5–1. Programmable circuits can be single-channel or multichannel. The programmable circuit (left) is a single-channel circuit with two memories, or programs. This means the trimmer settings for both programs can be adjusted by either a hand-held programmer or computer software. The listener can toggle between the two programs. One program might offer a more flat frequency response for listening in quiet, and the second program might offer less low-frequency gain and more high- frequency gain, which may be better for listening in background noise. The multichannel circuit (right) is available from some manufacturers in either a programmable or a nonprogrammable format. Again, the trimmer settings can be adjusted by a hand-held programmer or computer software. The multichannel circuit shown above has only one memory, meaning that the listener cannot adjust between or among different frequency responses.

set for difficult listening situations, such as when trying to hear speech with background noise. For this person, the program for listening in quiet might be set to provide the necessary gain that comes closest to meeting the target(s) of a fitting method. The other program might be set to provide less low-frequency gain and more high-frequency gain, which could enable better or more comfortable listening in noise. This might result in a reduction of low-frequency background noise and more gain for the normally less intense, high-frequency consonants of speech. Programmable hearing aids with more than one memory or pro-

Two Programmable Frequency Responses

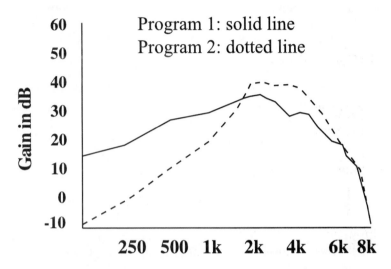

Figure 5–2. The response for Program 1 is set to most closely reach the target gain (for soft speech) for a hearing loss. Program 2 is set to enable "better", perhaps more comfortable, listening to speech in noise. Program 1 has broader, flatter frequency response than Program 2. Program 2 provides more gain for the high frequencies and less gain for the low frequencies than Program 1. Theoretically, this should make the high-frequency consonantal sounds of speech more audible and the "hubbub" of background noise less audible. The listener can voluntarily toggle between the two programs, depending on the listening situation.

gram (multi-memory) can be programmed to provide different clusters of trimmer settings for different listening situations.

An example of a single-channel programmable hearing aid is the Sigma™, by Unitron. It has six programmable trimmers: MPO, gain, low-cut tone control, high-cut tone control, compression kneepoint, and compression release time. These trimmer settings, when optimally programmed to meet a fitting method target(s), often compose Program 1. For program 2, an "X" (alternate gain) and a "Y" (alternate low-cut tone) trimmer can be programmed to provide a different frequency response. As shown in Figure 5–2, the alternate gain of Program 2 is set to provide more overall gain, which is supposed to increase audibility of the high-frequency consonants of speech. The alternate low-cut tone of Program 2 is set to provide less low-frequency gain, which is intended to decrease the audibility of background noise.

Multimemory hearing aids are not limited to providing different clusters of trimmer settings for different frequency responses. Different programmed memories can also provide alternate compression characteristics, or permit the client a choice between using directional versus omnidirectional microphone characteristics. The Audiozoom™ by Phonak is an example of a single-channel programmable hearing aid where the programmed memories each provide different microphone characteristics. One program serves to provide omnidirectional sound, while another program provides directional sound. As mentioned in Chapter 2, directional microphones are not a new development in the hearing aid industry, but they currently are definitely receiving a lot of attention.

Advantages of Programmable Hearing Aids

One advantage of programmable hearing aids is that access to all parameters (e.g., low-cut, high-cut, gain, MPO, compression kneepoint, etc.) can be obtained through the computer of the hand-held programmer. Not many ITEs will have a faceplate with more than three or four trimmers, because the "real estate," or space, on the faceplate may not accommodate more than this number. If changes in nonprogrammable trimmers are required, the clinician may need to return the hearing aid to the manufacturer. Completely different trimmer settings may be required, if, for example, a person's hearing loss fluctuates. It may also be that clients become accustomed to their hearing aids, and as such, their needs change. This might also prompt the clinician to change or "fine tune" the hearing aids. Programmability permits changes to any possible parameter or trimmer setting in the office, without the need to send the hearing aids back in to the manufacturer. A hand-held programmer allows easy access and is especially convenient when programming the hearing aids at the client's residence.

Another advantage of programmability is that it enables more interaction between clinician and client. Both visual and auditory feedback are available to clients when they can watch the programmed changes on the clinician's computer screen and at the same time can hear changes through the hearing aids. The visual input on the computer screen may also help to explain and illustrate the purpose and benefits of the hearing aids.

Computers are rapidly gaining acceptance in the public eye. Showing that hearing aid technology has kept in step with computer technology may also prompt clients to accept their hearing aids more readily.

DIGITAL HEARING AIDS

At this point, analog hearing aids (even those that are called "digitally programmable") are very different from true digital hearing aids. All hearing aids that do not have a digital circuit, or a DSP core, are analog hearing aids. Both analog and digital hearing aids share a microphone and a receiver, known as *transducers*. Transducers simply change energy from one form into another (microphones change sound into electricity and the receiver changes electricity back into sound). At the amplifier stage, gain is added to the input, and the sum total electrical current or voltage is sent on to the receiver, where it is converted back into sound. For hearing aids, the term *analog* means that the patterns of electrical current or voltages in the circuit are analogous (similar) to those of the acoustic (sound) input. The electrical voltages/current patterns are continuous (not discrete pieces), just like the incoming and outgoing sound waves. When thinking of analog, think about sound being played from old-time record albums on a stereo turntable. The needle wiggles in the grooves on the record, and these wiggle patterns are converted into analogous patterns of electricity, which are then amplified. These amplified patterns of electricity are then turned back into sound waves by the speakers (which are like microphones in reverse). Figure 5–3 shows a very simple schematic of an analog hearing aid circuit compared to that of a DSP hearing aid circuit. Note that the analog circuit includes two different kinds of energy: acoustic (i.e., sound) and electrical (i.e., voltage and current).

As Figure 5–3 shows, digital hearing aid has an additional transduction process; after the sound is transduced into electricity by the microphone, an analog-to-digital (A/D) converter changes the electrical current into binary sequences of numbers (or digits). These digits can be manipulated in almost any way possible to provide the gain or other digital processing instructions that are needed for someone's hearing requirements. Once the DSP algorithms have been executed (i.e., once the binary digits have been manipulated), the numbers are then changed back into electrical current by a digital-to-analog (D/A) converter, and this current is then transduced back into sound by the receiver.

When reading about DSP hearing aids, one may encounter the term "algorithm," which is simply a series of mathematical instructions. Numbers lend themselves easily to manipulation, and this ability is what makes DSP hearing aids very attractive. DSP circuitry allows even more complex processing than the already flexible analog, multichannel WDRC hearing aids (which were described in Chapter 4). With DSP, the frequency response can be literally "sculpted" to

Analog and Digital Hearing Aid Circuits

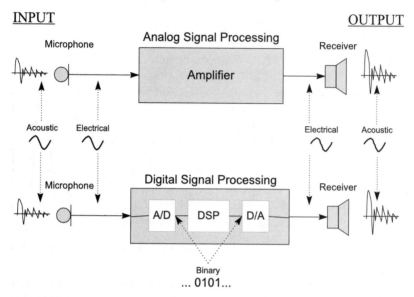

Figure 5–3. All hearing aid circuits (analog and digital) have a microphone and a receiver. The difference between the analog and the digital circuit is the processing that takes place between the microphone and the amplifier. In the analog circuit, there is a change from sound into electricity at the microphone; from there; the amplifier adds gain and at the receiver the sum total is changed back into sound. In the digital circuit, the microphone also changes sound into electricity and the analog-to-digital (A/D) converter changes the electricity into numbers. Here the gain is added (along with other elements of DSP). Past this point, the digital-to-analog (D/A) converter changes the numbers back into electricity and from there the receiver changes the electricity back into sound.

meet the target(s) of gain as closely as possible. Additional DSP algorithms provide other, unparalleled flexibility and adaptiveness not easily accomplished with analog circuitry. More advantages of DSP hearing aids are described later.

The basic thing to remember about DSP hearing aids is that sound is represented and manipulated by separate or discrete (not continuous) numbers or digits. When reading about DSP hearing aids, many terms are encountered: two of these are sampling rate and quantization. These refer to the way a digital circuit converts a continuous analog signal into a sequence of discrete numbers. In more simple terms, these terms refer to the way in which the frequency and the intensity of sound become represented by numbers. Figure 5-4 shows the basic

Sampling & Quantization

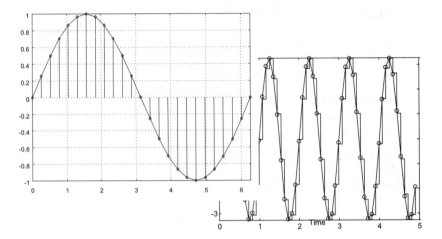

Figure 5–4. The graph on the left shows the incoming sound wave and how it becomes represented by numbers (digits) in a DSP hearing aid. A sound wave shows amplitude on the vertical axis, and time along the horizontal axis. Sampling rate of the DSP circuit is the frequency that the sound is represented with numbers (digits), and these are shown on the horizontal axis. The vertical lines on the left-most graph show the sound as it is sampled over time. If these lines were closer together, the sampling rate would be faster. Quantization of the DSP circuit represents intensity with numbers (digits), and these are shown on the vertical axis. The graph on the right shows the sound wave (on the left) as it represented digitally.

concepts behind sampling rate and quantization. The sampling rate is how often the digital circuit samples the amplitude of the analog signal, per some unit of time. In other words, the sampling rate is the frequency of sampling (seen as the horizontal axis of Figure 5-4). If the sampling rate is fast, these time between the samples taken is very small. A DSP circuit with a fast sampling rate, "samples" the sound more often as it changes over time than does a DSP circuit with a slower sampling rate. The higher the sampling rate, the greater the ability for the DSP circuit to accurately represent very high frequencies of sound with numbers. High frequencies have very short periods, or cycle times for each wavelength to occur. To represent these short wavelengths accurately with numbers requires a fast sampling rate that represents the sound over very small units of time.

Quantization is the ability of the DSP circuit to accurately represent the sound intensity (Figure 5–4, vertical axis). Quantization is the assigment of numbers to the samples of sound, where the numbers represent voltages or current levels. Quantization thus generates a stream or series of numbers that represent the sampled signal level. More quantization permits more accuracy of intensity representation by numbers. A sound wave that can be assigned, for example, 65,536 possible intensity values is far more accurately represented than the same sound wave when assigned, say, 256 possible intensity values. In the former cases, many different intensities can be assigned specific numerical value; in the latter case, intensities that are located between any one of the 256 possible values will have to be rounded up or down to the closest value. A high amount of quantization, thus, enables low distortion and a high dynamic range; this means very soft sounds as well as loud sounds can be captured or represented digitally. A high sampling rate together with many possible values for quantization, is like a fine-toothed comb: it permits a higher resolution or a more accurate numeric representation of the sound. Obviously, a high degree of quantization and a high sampling rate are preferred, but these may come with a cost—namely, high power consumption.

A complete discussion of DSP hearing aids is beyond the scope of this book; however, some concepts are roughly sketched here, along with some of the main ways in which they use compression. Several true digital hearing aids (i.e., those that have an actual DSP circuit) have recently come into the marketplace. The first DSP hearing aids were the Widex Senso™ and the Oticon DigiFocus™, which were released in 1996. Later, in 1997, Siemens introduced its Prisma™, and Philips and Resound introduced their DSP products. More models are being released as this book is being written. All of the four DSP hearing aids mentioned here are multichannel and programmable. The Widex Senso™ has three channels, and the Oticon DigiFocus™ has seven channels. The Siemens Prisma and Philips/Micro-Tech DSP hearing aids each have four channels.

Open Platform Versus Closed Platform

The terms open platform and closed platform are often used when describing DSP hearing aids and these refer to the degree to which the DSP hearing aids are software driven. A truly *open platform* DSP product would be similar to a regular computer; it would have hardware that would be able to run all kinds of software, from word processing to hearing aid compression characteristics. This would enable the freedom to provide whatever it takes to meet the needs of your client (Pavlovic,

Bisgaard, & Melanson, 1998). As yet, there are no such truly open platform DSP hearing aids.

An advantage of open platform DSP is that it enables complete flexibility, so that on any one hearing aid, totally different characteristics can be downloaded by software. On one open platform DSP hearing aid, completely different hearing aids could be created by software, from a linear, single-channel hearing aid to a two-channel WDRC hearing aid to a 10-channel hearing aid with input and output compression with multichannel WDRC. All parameters such as filters, directionality, MPO, and so on can be written in software (Edmonds, Staab, Preves, & Yanz, 1998). Disadvantages of a completely open platform DSP hearing aid is that, at this time, it has to be quite large and draw a lot of battery power; besides, the final end-product software might not be so very different from that used in closed platform DSP hearing aids (Kuk, 1998).

A *closed platform* DSP product has constraints built into the hardware that make the hearing aid dedicated to specific digital functions, such as having channels that represent bands of frequency. The digital functions inside the closed platform DSP hearing aid cannot be changed at will, because the hearing aid hardware itself is dedicated to performing certain functions. According to Kuk (1998), a closed platform DSP hearing aid is similar to an open platform DSP hearing aid, except that the manufacturer has elected to include in the hardware only portions necessary to provide benefit to the end user. As mentioned earlier, an advantage of closed platform is that the power consumption and size can be kept to a minimum. Both the Widex Senso™ and the Oticon DigiFocus™ are closed-platform DSP hearing aids.

Advantages of DSP Hearing Aids

The main advantage of DSP is that various compression schemes or combinations can be incorporated with increased flexibility and speed, without many of the constraints of analog circuits. One such analog constraint is the dB/octave slope between the channels. The steepest analog slope is 24 dB/octave (e.g., as available in Gennum's DynamEQ™ circuit, mentioned in Chapter 4). Although the 24 dB/octave slope permits a relative degree of independence between channels, it does not allow total independence. With DSP, the slope between adjacent channels can be almost infinitely steep compared to those of analog multichannel hearing aids. A very steep slope between channels permits an even higher degree of fitting flexibility for various shapes or configurations of hearing loss than that already obtained with the latest multichannel WDRC hearing aids.

Other advantages of DSP are that its complex numeric algorithms enable the ability to execute complex sets of commands, including: automatic noise reduction, directional microphones (see Chapter 2), feedback reduction, receiver peak equalization (cancellation of peaks in the frequency response), expansion (the opposite of compression) to reduce microphone noise, and so on. Noise reduction may make listening in noise more comfortable. Feedback reduction may be very helpful for the end user when using the telephone. By having the telephone close to the ear, any sound leaking from the receiver back to the microphone is actually enhanced, as it is literally guided to the microphone by bouncing off the telephone receiver. Receiver peak equalization is of value, because a smooth response may be more comfortable to the end user and may provide better sound quality. Both feedback reduction and receiver peak equalization might help to reduce the need for the screen-like filters that often become clogged by wax and other debris.

Expansion to reduce microphone noise, is a newcomer to the neighborhood of compression. Figure 5–5 shows the concept of expansion. Expansion, if seen on an input-output graph, would show a function or line that increases at an angle that is greater than 45° (left panel). The concept of expansion means that the hearing aid is providing even *more* than linear gain, and so, in this context, expansion is the opposite of compression. Note how it differs from WDRC, in that the output increases dramatically up until the kneepoint and then after the kneepoint, the pace slows down. The gain function (right panel) is shaped like a diamond; that is, the gain is not the same for all input levels below the kneepoint. Unlike WDRC, the greatest amount of gain is found only *at* the kneepoint of compression, and not for all input levels below the kneepoint. This implies that very soft sounds (around 10 to 20 dB input levels) are not given as much gain as 40 dB inputs.

The advantage of expansion is that it overcomes the problems noted by many clients who wear WDRC or the KAmp™; namely, that when there is some sounds around, the hearing aid sounds fine, but when things are very quiet in the environment, the hearing aid makes a "hiss" sound. This is especially noted by those who have relatively good low-frequency hearing. Some of this "hiss" in quiet comes from the amplification of internal microphone and circuit noise of the hearing aid. Because expansion provides very little gain for the very soft inputs, soft internal circuit and microphone noise is amplified very little. Expansion is well suited for DSP because it can be implemented with digital algorithms. In analog form, expansion may require large, more cumbersome, complicated circuitry.

With DSP, feedback reduction and receiver peak equalization can theoretically be accomplished in different ways: by reducing the gain

Expansion Versus WDRC

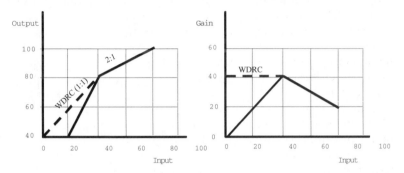

Some DSP hearing aids use expansion
•Reduces microphone noise in quiet
•Addresses typical noise complaint of K Amp & WDRC

Figure 5–5. The concept of expansion. Left, input-output graph shows function increasing at an angle of more than 45°. Right, the gain function using expansion.

in the channel where feedback or receiver peaks or is known to occur or by canceling the peaks where they occur by adding the same frequency and amplitude, but in an opposite phase.

The removal of background noise from speech has often been touted as a promising virtue of DSP. It should be mentioned here that an actual sampling and consequent removal or *subtraction* of background noise from speech is beyond what any DSP hearing aid can presently deliver. This is especially true if the background noise is not stationary, such as the babble of background speech. DSP hearing aids with a few channels can indeed sample stationary noise as being distinct from speech, but to separate and subtract fluctuating background noise would require many more channels than most DSP hearing aids (such as the Senso™ or DigFocus™) now employ. As mentioned in Chapter 2, speech is a rapidly fluctuating signal that varies constantly in amplitude, frequency, and time. To subtract background noise from speech would require many more than the two to four channels commonly used in hearing aids today, because the frequency regions where the speech and noise "collide" might be very narrow. A much "finer toothed comb" than is now feasible is necessary to attempt this fine an extraction. Furthermore, a sampling of speech and a sampling of noise would need to be employed at a high rate of units per second. Any noise that is sampled between the stops and starts of speech syllables could be extracted, but such a noise subtraction might at the same time also unintentionally remove some of the most important cues for distinguishing and categorizing elements of the target speech. The necessary DSP calculating power and speed to sample background speech babble from target speech cannot yet be readily housed in a small computer chip that would fit inside (or behind) someone's ear canal.

Present DSP technology does offer a more plausible solution to the problem of speech in background noise: namely, noise *reduction*, or *attenuation*. Noise reduction algorithms in DSP are complicated but the broad strokes of the basics are not that hard to grasp. Essentially, an "algorithm" is just a series of instructions, like "go two steps forward, then go one step back, then three steps forward, and so on. Noise reduction algorithms assume that noise is more stationary in intensity than the speech that someone is trying to hear; that is, the speech right in front of you is bound to rise and fall in intensity more than the ongoing hubbub of background noise, be it speech or an air conditioner. DSP essentially looks at whether the intensity of the incoming sound fluctuates or not (see Figure 5–6). If the sound intensity is stationary or stable, the noise reduction algorithm determines that the sound is noise. If the sound fluctuates past a certain point, the noise reduction algorithm ascertains that the sound is speech. In other words, noise reduction algorithms are like an artificial intelligence that looks at the statistical distribution of sound input intensities to determine if the sound is noise or speech. If the sound is determined to be speech in one or more channels of the DSP hearing aid, then the gain is maintained. If the sound is determined to be noise, then the gain in the channel where the noise is sensed is reduced. It must be remembered, however, that reducing the gain in any channel reduces both the background noise and the speech cues. This can be accomplished more readily with DSP than with analog hearing aids, because DSP hearing aids can actively reduce the gain in channels where the background noise is most present. These are just some of the advantages of DSP, but in the long run, these may go a long way to provide comfort as well as audibility for the end user. DSP hearing aids can also provide a notoriously *clean sound* to the end user, without the internal amplifier noise commonly associated with some analog circuitry.

Regarding DSP and speech performance in the midst of background noise, there are important but very different roles that noise reduction algorithms and directional microphones each tend to serve. So far, precious little data are available to show that noise reduction actually improves the intelligibility of speech while listening in background noise. However, many *subjective* comments of increased comfort in background noise, are given by clients who have experienced noise reduction with their DSP hearing aids. On the other hand, directional microphones have in-

Noise Reduction Algorithms
Used In Some DSP Hearing Aids

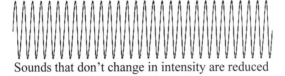

Sounds that don't change in intensity are reduced

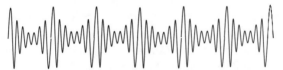

Sounds that change in intensity are not reduced

Figure 5–6. DSP hearing aid using a noise reduction algorithm.

deed been shown to *objectively* increase the listening performance while listening in background noise (see Chapter 2). Perhaps this is why many manufacturers are recognizing the twin-headed endeavor to include in their latest DSP products (1) noise reduction algorithms, for subjective comfort, and (2) directional microphones, for objective listening performance. So far, the Siemens Prisma™ and ReSound DSP products incorporate both noise reduction algorithms and directional microphones. Others are sure to follow.

Two Examples of Digital Hearing Aids

The salient features of the two earliest DSP (closed platform) hearing aids should be mentioned before leaving the discussion of DSP because they are receiving a lot of attention. They are also very different from each other. The Widex Senso™ has three channels with adjustable cross-over frequency controls (to be discussed more in Chapter 6), which adjust the frequency where adjacent channels "meet." Cross-over controls enable the channels to be widened or narrowed. The gain can be adjusted separately for each channel, depending on the shape of the hearing loss (where it rises or falls). Each channel has compression that is geared to accomplish normal loudness growth for the listener (WDRC).

An interesting aspect of the Senso™ is that the threshold kneepoint of compression can be set to as low as 15–20 dB SPL. In the Senso™, this low kneepoint is associated with an exceptionally large amount of gain for low-intensity input sounds. With analog hearing aids, this low knee-point is not normally utilized because excessive feedback would be generated by the large amount of gain applied to the low-intensity input sounds.

The attack/release times of the Senso™ are several hundreds of milliseconds in length; these relatively long dynamic characteristics are similar to those provided by AVC (see Chapter 4). Long attack/release times are employed by the Senso™, because shorter attack/release times combined with the low kneepoint of compression were not well received by many initial users. The dynamic aspects of compression remain relatively slow in a stationary noise environment, but they will speed up if a sudden, intense transient sound occurs (Ludvigsen, 1997).

During the initial fitting of the Senso™, audiometry is used to determine hearing thresholds by emitting complex tones from the hearing aid while it is in the ear of the listener. These are used to determine targets for gain. The advantage of this method is that the results include the effects of the earmold or the shell of the hearing aid in situ (in place) in the ear.

The Senso™ uses an ongoing statistical method separately in each of its three channels, whereby every few seconds, the speech and background noise are sampled. The properties of single-talker speech are sampled as being statistically more variable in intensity than the more stationary, consistent intensity of background speech noise babble. This difference is used to determine in which frequency band most background noise is present. An assumption is also made that in loud listening situations, speech is also spoken louder (Ludvigsen, 1997). When a channel senses that background noise is present, the gain for both the speech and the noise is reduced in that channel. Because speech in noise is normally spoken at a more intense level, the speech is still assumed to be audible.

Oticon's DigiFocus™ has seven channels (Oticon prefers to call them frequency bands), with each band representing a range of audiometric frequencies. Unlike those of the Widex Senso™, the cross-over frequencies of the DigiFocus™ cannot be adjusted; that is, bands that are adjacent to each other cannot be widened or narrowed. Despite being fixed in place, the seven bands each represent a relatively narrow range of frequencies, which permits a high degree of fitting flexibility for people who have difficult-to-fit hearing loss configurations. An interesting feature of the DigiFocus™ fitting strategy is the separation of the seven bands into low and high frequency ranges (a low-frequency channel composed of three low-frequency bands and a high-frequency channel composed of four high-frequency bands).

Central to the Oticon DigiFocus™ philosophy is the concept of "adaptive speech alignment," which is intended to address the complexities of aiding the acoustic signal of speech. The goal of this philosophy is to provide aided speech that is as intelligible as possible. To achieve this goal, the DigiFocus™ does not provide a proprietary noise reduction algorithm or strategy, like that of the Widex Senso™. The DigiFocus™ concentrates, instead, on accurate and specific frequency shaping with its seven bands; it also provides very different attack/release times for the low-frequency and high-frequency channels.

The low-frequency channel provides WDRC, along with syllabic compression (fast attack/release times). The high-frequency channel provides output limiting compression, along with slower acting attack/release times (what Oticon calls "adaptive gain"). Consistent with output limiting (described in Chapter 4), the gain for the high-frequency channel is essentially linear over a wide range of input levels, with a high kneepoint and high compression ratio to limit the output from exceeding the listener's UCLs. The attack times for the high-frequency channel are about 20 ms, with release times that vary from about 230 ms to 320 ms.

Think of the soft, high-frequency, unvoiced consonants of speech as fragile china teacups and think of the louder, low-frequency vowels of speech as bulls in a china shop. The bulls, if unchecked, would smash everything in sight. In the same way, the vowels, through the upward spread of masking (see Chapter 1) would threaten to cover up the fragile, high-frequency consonants.

The syllabic compression for the low-frequency channel is designed to reduce the upward spread of masking of low-frequency vowels (generally more intense speech sounds), which can obliterate the audibility of high-frequency consonantal speech (generally less intense speech sounds). Recall from Chapter 4, that the attack/release times of syllabic compression are intended to be shorter in duration that the average syllable of speech, which will presumably reduce the differences between the normally more intense voiced vowels and the softer unvoiced consonants. The hoped-for result is a more uniform aided intensity for all speech sounds for the listener who wears the hearing aids, so that the hearing aid makes the softer consonantal sounds of speech more audible without simultaneously making the normally louder vowel portions of speech too loud.

DSP: State of the Art and the Future

One thing that is evident about the various available DSP products is that the manufacturers are highly secretive about the specific methods they use. This is understandable, considering the highly competitive nature of the DSP market. Each manufacturer has developed their own type of DSP circuit that also contains very specific algorithms. Unlike typical analog hearing aids, which are built from parts that are often available to any manufacturer, DSP hearing aids are very proprietary in their composition. As mentioned earlier, only the microphone and receivers in DSP hearing aids can be similar to those of analog hearing aids. The actual DSP circuit core is quite unique to any one specific DSP product. To release details of an actual proprietary DSP circuit core to the general arena of hearing aid manufacturing would be giving away what probably took a lot of time and money to develop.

On the other hand, some clinicians have been frustrated over what they see as an inability to access or measure when fitting DSP hearing aids. The DSP products are, in some ways, like closed boxes: the manufacturer may know what is going on inside the hearing aid, but the clinician has no choice but to trust that the fitting will be satisfactory for clients. Many terms relating specifically to individual DSP products (such as, "adaptive gain") are not readily understandable, because they are used nowhere else. The bottom line is that clients are, indeed, often highly satisfied with their DSP hearing aids, noting that they are an improvement from their old analog hearing aids. The clinician, however, is not always very sure why this is true.

A challenge for the future of DSP hearing aids is to continue to create smaller and smaller DSP circuits. The physical size of DSP circuits has been larger than most analog circuits, and the size is often measured in "microns." At this time, DSP circuits are often 0.2 to 0.3 microns in size, which means a digital CIC can be very challenging to make. If DSP circuits can be reduced in size to less than 0.2 microns, then building CIC versions of DSP hearing aids will be a lot more feasible.

SUMMARY

■ Digitally programmable and digital hearing aids are not the same and cannot be referred to interchangeably. The term "digitally programmable" simply means the hearing aid trimmers and VC can be adjusted by software or by a hand-held programming device. Some analog and all digital hearing aids can be programmed and, thus, can be considered "programmable." The term "digitally programmable" means the hearing aid can be programmed by a computer, which is itself digital. A truly digital hearing aid circuit, like a computer, runs on binary sequences of 0's and 1's, or digits.

■ Programmable hearing aids can be single-channel or multi-channel. Most programmable hearing aids have more than one memory or program, so that the listener can voluntarily toggle between them for optimal listening in different listening situations. Some programmable hearing aids usually have a single program, meaning that the trimmers can be accessed and set via a computer or hand-held programming unit, but the listener cannot toggle between different programs. 3M (ReSound) has a patent for an analog, multichannel, multiprogram hearing aid.

■ Digital hearing aids change sound into numerical or digital information. These digits can be manipulated at will, by long sets of commands, called "algorithms." The fact that digits can be manipulated in almost any conceivable way, is what makes is what makes DSP hearing aids more flexible and adaptive to different listening environments than their analog counterparts.

RECOMMENDED READING

Edmonds, J., Staab, W. J., Preves, D., & Yanz, J. (1997). "Open" digital hearing aids: A reality today. *The Hearing Journal, 50*(10), 54–56.

Kuk, F. K., (1997). Open or closed? Let's weigh the evidence. *The Hearing Journal, 50*(10), 54–56.

Ludvigsen, C. (1997, March). Basic amplification rationale of a DSP hearing instrument. *The Hearing Review.*

Pavlovic. C., Bisgaard, N., & Melanson, J. (1997). The next step: "Open" digital hearing aids. *The Hearing Journal, 50*(5), 65–66.

Schum, D. J. (1998). Open digital platforms: Opportunities and responsibilities. *The Hearing Journal, 51*(1), 44–46.

CHAPTER 6

Expanding On Compression

This chapter expands what was discussed and poses further questions. Two main concepts should be apparent from the last five chapters: namely (1) the cochlea is an active organ in hearing and (2) hearing aids are being designed and used to imitate the functions of the cochlea. Perhaps two more things have also become more obvious: (1) we have come a long distance in hearing aid design and (2) we still have to cover much more distance to achieve hearing aid sound transparency.

HEARING AIDS AND THE TRAVELING WAVE REVISITED

The different roles of the IHCs and OHCs were compared in Chapter 1. The IHCs send virtually all sound information to the brain, but incoming sounds below 40 to 50 dB sound pressure level (SPL) will not create a traveling wave large enough to stimulate the IHCs. The OHCs, with their stretching/shrinking mechanical motion, affect the motion of the basilar membrane so the IHCs can sense these soft sounds. The OHCs also sharpen the peak of the traveling wave, which otherwise is rounded and dull.

Hearing aids cannot truly restore normal cochlear function, because they cannot replace damaged or missing hair cells. Hearing aids can only manipulate one independent variable, amplification. Making sounds louder, however, even with compression, does not sharpen the peak of the traveling wave. Hearing aids can, however, work toward the imitation of OHC function along one dimension; (i.e., they can specifically amplify soft input sounds more than intense input sounds). This is the purpose behind wide dynamic range compression (WDRC).

This admission of cochlear humility does, however, bring up a challenge for hearing aid design of the future. Could hearing aids approximate a more real imitation of OHC function if they somehow sharpened the peak of the traveling wave while they amplified sound?

Is it possible for future digital hearing aids (see Chapter 5) to somehow sharpen the incoming sound waves so they create a sharper traveling wave in the damaged cochlea? (see Figure 6–1). If this could be done, hearing aids *could* step beyond the present, simple focus of WDRC, and truly imitate the function of healthy outer hair cells. Such a hearing aid might sound strange to the person with normal hearing, but maybe it would sound good, and really help speech recognition in noisy situations, for the person with mild-to-moderate SNHL. But would sharpened sound waves actually translate into sharpened traveling waves in the cochlea?

The aforesaid implies sharpening sound waves, but perhaps it might be helpful to look at sharpening along another dimension: the spectrum.

A Possible DSP Issue for the Future
Spectral Sharpening

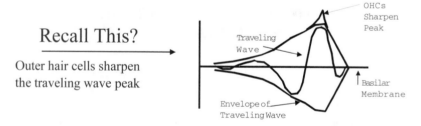

Recall This?

Outer hair cells sharpen
the traveling wave peak

What if we tried this?

Why not sharpen the peaks
of input sounds?

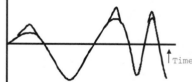

Figure 6–1.

Here it is necessary to consider the two ways in which sound is common-ly represented (see Figure 6–2). Sound takes place in three dimensions: frequency, intensity, and time. Sound waves depict sound in terms of in-tensity (amplitude) and time. Amplitude of sound is shown as vertical fluctuations that take place over time, seen on the horizontal plane. The peaks that appear in a sound wave represent energy at specific frequen-cies. To sharpen or otherwise exaggerate these peaks requires either an en-hancement of the peak itself or else a reduction of the sound energy around the peak. This implies a deliberate shaping or sculpting of sound.

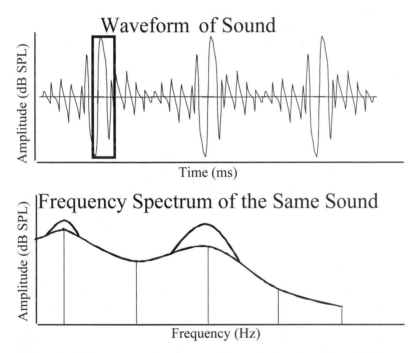

Figure 6–2. The figure shows two ways of depicting a sound. The top shows a time waveform of a periodic sound (the cycles repeat over time), which means it is tonal in quality. It is a complex sound, composed of more than one pure tone. The peaks of greatest amplitude are visible, but the frequency where the most amplitude occurs is not easy to determine. The bottom shows a frequency spec-trum of the same sound. The spectrum is a "slice" taken from a section (within the box) of the sound wave on top. In a spectrum, the frequency peaks where the most amplitude occurs is readily evident; in this example, the lowest frequency component of the complex sound has the greatest amplitude, and the highest fre-quency component has the least amplitude. Time, however, cannot be seen on a frequency spectrum. There are advantages to both ways of depicting a sound; it all depends on what information is required.

Sound sharpening also can be explained in terms of a *frequency spectrum*, which shows of amplitude on the vertical axis and frequency on the horizontal axis (see Figure 6–1). Unlike the sound wave, in the frequency spectrum, the dimension of time is missing. On the other hand, the frequency of a sound wave can only be computed indirectly. The relationship of a frequency spectrum to a sound wave is like that of a single "slice" from a loaf of bread. The spectrum is like the slice of bread pulled out of the loaf and turned around flat to face the one who will eat it.

If the peak of the sound wave is shown on a spectral "slice," the energy of specific frequencies at and around the peak can be readily identified. These frequencies can be specifically enhanced and this is what is known as the "spectral sharpening" of sound. A hearing aid circuit can theoretically both sharpen and amplify sound to be delivered to the eardrum. Perhaps the end product would sound rather "sharp" or piercing to the person with a normal-hearing ear, but would it sound good to the person with OHC damage?

This has got to be easier said than done or else it would have been already done. As a matter of fact, spectral sharpening has been tried with analog technology (Stone & Moore, 1992); however, it did not meet with much success. According to Stone and Moore (1992), the spectrum of speech in background noise shows that the "valleys" between the peaks of speech are filled with noise. Those with SNHL have a more difficult time discerning the peaks of speech from the valleys filled with noise and, therefore, are greatly affected by background noise when trying to listen to speech. As mentioned in Chapters 1 and 2, we normally require speech to be at least as intense (or 2.5 dB more intense) as background noise to understand 50% of the speech (Killion, 1998); those with SNHL require an additional 5 dB of speech compared to the noise to understand 50% of the speech. Furthermore, each additional 1 dB of speech (in relation to the level of he background noise) results in roughly a 10% increase in speech intelligibility.

In their experiment, Stone and Moore (1992) used an analog filterbank composed of 16 frequency bands or channels. For speech input sounds, various channels among the 16 were used to increase the intensity of the sound peaks, depending on the their frequency locations. A total of 10 subjects with mild-to-moderate SNHL were then tested for their speech reception ability in the presence of continuous background noise. In one experiment, subjects wore their own hearing aids, most of which were linear. The background noise was presented at two different levels (44 and 64 dB SPL), and the speech was presented at a level that was 3 dB more intense than these background noise levels. In another experiment, the subjects did not wear their hearing aids; instead, the stimuli were given high-frequency emphasis so as to imitate the function of their own hearing aids. In the second experiment, the subjects adjusted the level of the background noise to match levels they normally found to be comfortable in their everyday lives. Speech intelligibility did not improve for Stone and Moore's subjects, and in some case, it even became worse. The second experiment, however, showed that they did have a *subjective* impression that speech stood out better against background noise. The article by Stone and Moore (1992) is quite technical, and the interested reader is encouraged to examine it for further details.

As mentioned in Chapter 2, the obstacles to better reception of speech in noise are considerable. The removal of background noise from speech is easier to accomplish, if the background noise is stationary (i.e., not fluctuating) in nature. It is also much easier for any available circuit (analog or digital) to spectrally sharpen the peaks a steady-state, continuous pure tone than it is to do the same for complex, quickly changing sounds, like speech. Even the new digital hearing aids do not now achieve spectral sharpening as outlined in Stone and Moore's (1992) experiment.

Even if incoming sound waves can be successfully honed to create a sharpened traveling wave, this may still not help people with missing or damaged IHCs. Recall that IHC damage may be a cause of especially poor discrimination of speech in noise (Chapter 1).

COMMON CLINICAL COMBINATIONS OF COMPRESSION

Some common combinations of compression are often encountered by clinicians. Although there are no absolute maxims calling for the endorsement of one type of compression over another for various clinical populations, there are, however, some trends, as described here.

Three dimensions of compression were woven together in Chapter 4: (1) output versus input compression, (2) conventional compression controls versus the TK control, and (3) output limiting compression versus WDRC. These six aspects of compression are often found together in two predictable compression combinations, and each one can serve a different clinical population (see Figure 6–3).

A Compression Combination for Severe-to-Profound Hearing Loss

Output compression and output limiting compression work well together in the same circuit. This combination has several features for clients with severe-to-profound hearing loss. Severe-to-profound hearing loss usually results in a small dynamic range (i.e., about 20 dB) and protection

Summary: Applying Compression

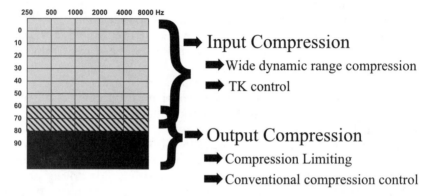

Figure 6–3. WDRC, which is a type of input compression, is well suited for fitting mild-to-moderate SNHL. Output limiting, which is almost always used with output compression circuits, is suited for fitting severe-to-profound hearing losses. The diagonal lines in the range from 60 to 80 dB hearing losses, represents a "gray" area of intersection for the fitting of either type of hearing aid.

of residual hearing is critical for these clients. With output compression, the client can be assured that although the volume controls of these hearing aids change the kneepoint of compression, they affect only the gain and *not* the MPO. Independent from the VC, a conventional compression control in the hearing aid also changes the compression kneepoint, and this adjusts the MPO. The output limiting compression in the hearing aid means that the compression kneepoint occurs at a relatively high input level, along with a high ratio or degree of compression. If the hearing aid has a high-power circuit, the client receives lots of linear gain for soft to at least conversational speech input levels, but once the output comes close to the individual's loudness tolerance levels, the hearing aid provides a high degree of compression to limit the output. Although normal loudness growth has not been achieved for these clients, they do get a strong degree of amplification and an output that is limited without the distortion of linear peak clipping.

A Compression Combination for Mild-to-Moderate Hearing Loss

Input compression and WDRC also work well together in the same circuit. This combination has several features for clients with mild-to-moderate SNHL. Mild-to-moderate hearing loss usually results in a relatively larger dynamic range of 40 to 60 dB. With input compression, the VC does not affect the kneepoint of compression, but it does affect the gain and the MPO together. A TK control changes the kneepoint of compression, and it also specifically affects the gain for soft incoming sounds. Recall from Chapter 4, that in hearing aids with the TK control, the gain for soft input sounds is *increased* as the kneepoint is lowered. The WDRC in the hearing aid means that the kneepoint of compression occurs at a relatively low input level, along with a low ratio or degree of compression. WDRC hearing aids usually have a medium power circuit, which means the client receives linear gain for only very soft input levels. The hearing aid is otherwise in a low degree of compression over a wide range of input levels. With these features clients get a greater degree of amplification for soft input sounds and less amplification for sounds that are well within their dynamic range. Recall from Chapters 2 and 3, that for these clients, the "floor" of hearing sensitivity is raised, while the "ceiling" of loudness tolerance is similar to that of normal hearing.

Input compression with WDRC is applicable to the largest clinical population (i.e., those persons with mild-to-moderate SNHL). It is, therefore, very important to categorize it properly. Input compression with WDRC can be further subdivided into two more subsets: bass increases at low levels (BILL) and treble increases at low levels (TILL). As mentioned in Chapter 4, BILL and TILL are two types or subsets of WDRC, and WDRC is a type or subset of input compression. Recall that BILL hearing aids offer most compression for the low frequencies and TILL offers most compression for the high frequencies. A straight WDRC hearing aid that is neither BILL nor TILL offers a more similar degree of compression across the frequencies.

A visual categorization of input compression is shown in Figure 6–4. WDRC is a type of input compression, but not all input compression is WDRC. Similarly, BILL and TILL are two types of WDRC, but not all WDRC is specifically BILL or TILL. The K Amp™ hearing aid, which is TILL, is a type of WDRC, which in turn is also a type of input compression. The Oticon Multifocus™ hearing aid, which is BILL, is also WDRC, which in turn is again, a type of input compression.

As mentioned in Chapter 4, the DynamEQII™ is a two-channel WDRC circuit from the Gennum Corporation that effectively combines BILL and TILL in one hearing aid. The low-frequency channel offers BILL and the high-frequency channel offers TILL. This circuit has been available to many hearing aid manufacturers for the past few years. Other manufacturers have designed their own multichannel WDRC circuits that can provide a similar degree of fitting flexibility.

A big advantage of the multichannel circuit over a single-channel WDRC circuit involves clinical fitting flexibility. Either the BILL or

Categorizing Input Compression

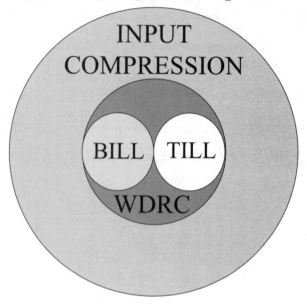

Figure 6–4. Because input compression can be applied to a large segment of the hearing aid fitting population, clinicians may find some categorization helpful. As shown, all WDRC is input compression, but not all input compression is WDRC. Input compression that is not WDRC probably has compression kneepoints and ratios that are more like those of output limiting compression. Bass increases and treble increases at low levels (BILL and TILL) are WDRC, but not all WDRC is BIL or TILL. Some WDRC is neither BILL nor TILL; for WDRC that is neither BILL nor TILL, low inputs result in an equal amount of gain increase at all frequencies.

TILL channel can be turned up or down to provide an optimal fitting for particular configurations or shapes of mild-to-moderate hearing loss. In essence, only one hearing aid circuit may be required to fit many different hearing losses. Because of the preponderance of presbycusis and other types of mild-to-moderate SNHL, the flexible multichannel WDRC circuits can potentially be fit on many people.

AN EXAMPLE OF MULTICHANNEL WDRC: UNITRON'S "SOUND FX"

Due to the recent popularity of multichannel WDRC hearing aids, it may be helpful to illustrate an example of such a hearing aid from one hearing aid manufacturer. The Sound FX™ by Unitron Industries Ltd. is an example of a two-channel WDRC hearing aid that offers BILL and TILL together in one hearing aid. As mentioned in Chapter 4, it is built on the DynamEQII™ circuit by Gennum Corporation. The Sound FX™ can be adjusted to provide BILL, TILL, or both, which permits a high degree of fitting flexibility. Some unique features of the Sound FX™ and its controls or trimmers are described briefly here. Many of these can also be found on hearing aids by other manufacturers that have used the DynamEQII™ circuit.

Steep dB/Octave Slope Between the Channels

The DynamEQII™ circuit allows for a 12 dB/octave slope or a more steep 24 dB/octave slope between its two channels. The Sound FX™ uses the more steep 24 dB/octave slope (see Figure 6–5). The term "slope" for a multi-channel hearing aid refers to the steepness of the "sides" or "skirts" of the channels. Both channels of the Sound FX™ provide gain over a range of frequencies, and at the cross-over frequency region where the two channels "meet," the gain of each channel decreases by a rate of 24 dB/octave.

Fitting Flexibility

For analog (nondigital) technology, 24 dB/octave is a relatively steep slope that contributes to the fitting flexibility of the Sound FX™. Fitting flexibility is further enhanced when the cross-over frequency between the two channels can be adjusted. The Sound FX™ has an F control that adjusts the frequency crossover point where the channels come together. Probe microphone, or "real ear," measures of ear canal sound pressure levels reveal that the F control can be used to adjust the frequency crossover from about 500 Hz to about 2000 Hz.

Fitting flexibility is maximized when the gain of the low and high channels can be adjusted independently, along with the crossover frequency. In the Sound FX™, the gain of the low-frequency channel (GL control) can be turned up without affecting the frequency regions of the high-frequency channel; similarly, the gain of the high-frequency channel (GH control) can be turned up without affecting the frequency regions of the low-frequency channel. It is thus as if there are two "vertical" gain controls and a "horizontal" cross-over control.

These three controls enable fitting of difficult hearing loss configurations (e.g., the "reverse" hearing loss where the client has hearing loss for the low frequencies and better hearing for the high frequencies or the precipitous hearing loss where the hearing is normal up to 2000

A Two-Channel Hearing Aid
with a Steep Slope Between Channels

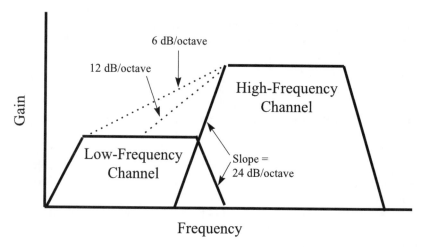

Figure 6–5. "Passive" low-cut or high-cut trimmers usually have a 6 dB/octave slope. "Active" trimmers have a 12 or 18 dB/octave slope, which enables them to have more dramatic effects on the frequency response. A steep 24 dB/octave slope between two channels of a hearing aid enables independence between the channels, and consequently, even more flexibility in shaping the frequency response. It also helps to eliminate unwanted mid-frequency gain when this is desired (e.g., when fitting hearing losses that suddenly drop or improve). Two channels divided by a steep slope provide low- and high-frequency "plateaus," that can be raised or lowered with low-frequency and high channel gain trimmers. In this example, the low-frequency channel gain is turned down while the high-frequency gain is turned up.

Hz, and then suddenly drops off in the high frequencies). When fitting precipitous high-frequency hearing losses with single-channel hearing aids, gain for the high frequencies is typically provided, along with a maximum degree of low-cut. A common problem, however, is unavoidable and unwanted gain for the mid-frequencies where the person may have no hearing loss. The fitting flexibility of the Sound FX™ and similar two-channel devices enables the frequency response to be "sculpted" around the "corner" in the audiogram.

Adjustable Compression Ratios

The clinician should know that for the Sound FX™, an adjustment of the GL (gain for low channel) and GH (gain for high channel) controls is really an adjustment of the compression *ratios*. Input/output graphs show that for each channel, the Sound FX™ has two kneepoints and adjustable compression ratios (see Figure 6–6). This feature is very useful for restoring normal loudness growth. The two-channel DynamEQII™ circuit is by no means the only circuit that has these features. In fact, Re-Sound, Inc. has long been known for restoring normal loudness growth by means of a WDRC circuit with two kneepoints and adjustable compression ratios.

Figure 6–6 illustrates how the concepts of compression kneepoints and ratios are related to the restoration of normal loudness growth. The right side shows the reduced dynamic range and abnormal loudness growth that occurs with sensorineural hearing loss. It also shows the required gain to restore normal loudness growth. The smaller dy-

Loudness Growth
&
Compression Ratios

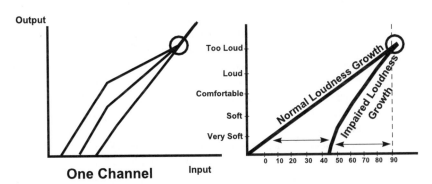

Figure 6–6. The relationship of the concepts of loudness growth and compression ratios are shown. In the right graph, the right arrow shows the dynamic range for someone's HL at some frequency; the left arrow shows required gain to restore normal loudness growth. The circle shows the "ceiling" of loudness tolerance for both SNHL and normal hearing. On the left is an input/output graph for one channel of the two-channel DynamEQII™ circuit; the circle shows the second, higher kneepoint that corresponds to the "ceiling" of loudness tolerance on the right. The diagonal lines rising from the X axis show the linear gain below the kneepoint of compression, which is adjusted by a TK control. The compression ratios hinge the second, higher kneepoint. The lines sloping to the left of the second kneepoint show the adjustable ratios of compression needed to restore normal loudness growth.

namic range will require a greater amount of gain to restore normal loudness growth.

The left side of Figure 6–6 shows an input/output graph that features two kneepoints and adjustable compression ratios. It can represent any one channel of the DynamEQII™ circuit. The lower kneepoint shows the input SPL where compression "begins." Below this input level, the gain is linear. A TK control adjusts this lower kneepoint for both channels together; the Sound FX™ thus has only one TK control. Between the two kneepoints, the compression ratio can range from 4:1 to 1:1 (which is WDRC). Note that the compression ratios "hinge" from the *second, higher* kneepoint, not from the first lower kneepoint. With this in mind, it becomes clear that as the compression ratio increases, so does the gain! This is contrary to most other types of compression, in which an increased compression ratio is associated with decreased gain.

The higher kneepoint shows where compression "ends." Beyond this input SPL, the hearing aid has reached a point of "unity gain." Here, the compression ratio once again becomes linear, but there is no gain whatsoever. For example, a 95 dB input results in a 95 dB output, a 96 dB input results in a 96 dB output, and so on. It is at this point that the hearing aid becomes truly acoustically "transparent."

The two-channel DynamEQII™ (in this case, the Sound FX™) feature of adjustable compression ratios separately for both channels is a strong tool for restoring normal loudness growth. With increased compression ratio (increased gain), there is an approximation toward the ideal of restoring normal loudness growth. The TK control, at one time the only control available to adjust the compression of WDRC hearing aids, can now be relegated to a more "rear seat" in the theater. When it comes to restoring normal loudness growth, adjusting compression ratios is a stronger tool than adjusting compression kneepoints (see left graph of Figure 6–6).

Adjustment of the kneepoint and ratios, however, should be seen as two parts of a team. The GL and GH controls, which adjust compression ratio, should be set to best restore normal loudness growth for the client. In general, if the client's dynamic range is one-fourth that of normal for some frequency range, then adjust the compression ratio to 4:1 (the maximum gain position for either the GL of the GH control). If the client's dynamic range is half that of normal, then adjust the compression ratio so it is 2:1. Specific compression ratios for specific GL or GH control positions should be provided by the manufacturer.

The TK control should be adjusted to provide as much gain for soft input sounds as possible, without at the same time resulting in feedback or the client's perception of a background "hiss." Recall from Chapter 4 that the TK control at a "minus" position lowers the kneepoint of compression and increases the gain for soft input sounds. Setting the TK at a "plus" position raises the kneepoint and reduces the effectiveness of the WDRC.

Fitting Multichannel WDRC: Case Studies

Several examples of flexible multi-channel WDRC hearing aids fittings (all of them with the Sound FX™, based on the Gennum DynamEQII™ circuit) are shown in the next five figures (Figures 6–7 through 6–11). Figure 6–7 is an example of a fitting for a person with bilateral, mild-to-

Case #1: Noise Exposure, Presbycusis
First hearing aid fitting (Sound FX canals, MPO 100 dB SPL)

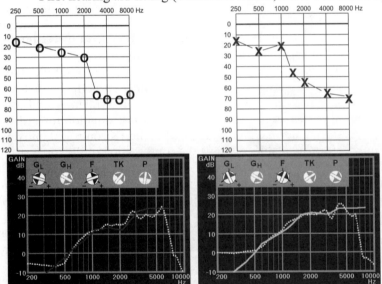

Figure 6–7. The results shown are from the right and left ears of a person with presbycusis and a history of noise exposure. The real ear measures shown (with NAL-R targets) are obtained from the Sound FX™ (ITE style) by Unitron. The input level was 50 dB SPL. The results are from one of my first fittings of analog, multi-channel WDRC hearing aids (nonprogrammable). The trimmers settings used are shown in the top of the real ear measurements (bottom panels). The darker trimmers appeared on the faceplate as screwdriver controls; the lighter trimmers are preset, and built into the hearing aids. The insertion gain (dotted lines) are close to meeting the NAL-R targets (solid lines) for both ears.

moderate SNHL. The ITE (canal style) hearing aids provide insertion gain that comes close to meeting the NAL-R targets for both ears. Note from the figure, that the gain for the low frequencies is turned toward "minus," while the gain for the high frequencies is turned toward "plus." The frequency cross-over control is positioned between one-half and "plus" for both ears, indicating that the cross-over frequency between the two channels is set between 1000 and 2000 Hz.

The same hearing aid circuit (ITE canal style) was measured on a person with a monaural "reverse" SNHL (Figure 6–8), which demonstrates the flexibility of the Gennum DynamEQII™ circuit. Again, the insertion gain comes quite close to meeting the NAL-R target for this hearing loss. Usually, reverse hearing losses are notoriously difficult to fit because most hearing aids provide more gain for the high frequencies than they do for the low frequencies. In this case, the insertion gain matches the target most closely for the low to mid frequencies; the gain

Case #2: Sudden Hearing Loss After Car Accident

Diagnosed as having endolymphatic hydrops
Client's second hearing aid fitting
Monaural Sound FX Canal, MPO 110 dB SPL)

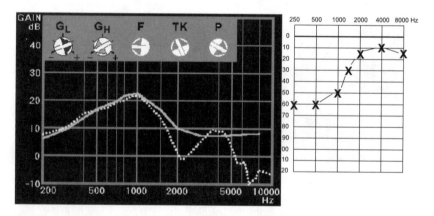

Figure 6–8. This person has a "reverse" hearing loss, and is wearing the same type of hearing aid as the person in Figure 6–6 (Sound FX™ by Unitron, canal style). Note the flexibility of this analog, multichannel WDRC hearing aid; in this case, it comes close to meeting the real ear NAL-R target for a 50 dB input sound level. There is a gap between the insertion gain (dotted line) and the target (solid line) around 2000 Hz; however, for reverse hearing losses, the usual difficulty is in meeting low-frequency targets without exceeding high-frequency targets.

drops below target around 2000 Hz, probably because there is a loss of the person's natural ear canal resonance when it is occluded by the hearing aid (real ear aided response minus real ear unaided response equals real ear insertion response, or gain). The gain for the high frequencies, however, does actually "recuperate" and it once again close to the NAL-R target.

Figure 6–9 shows the fitting results for a person with a monaural, precipitous high-frequency hearing loss; this time, however, the circuit was a programmable version of the Gennum DynamEQII and it was housed inside a CIC-style of shell. The insertion gain again closely matches the NAL-R insertion gain target; however, when the same programmed trimmer settings were measured according to the DSL fitting method, the output falls below the DSL targets.

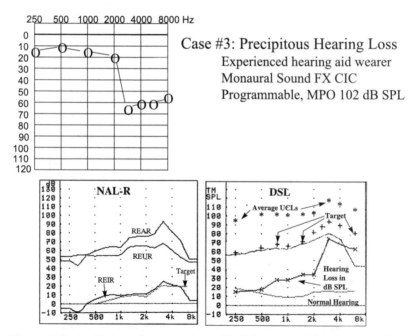

Case #3: Precipitous Hearing Loss
Experienced hearing aid wearer
Monaural Sound FX CIC
Programmable, MPO 102 dB SPL

Figure 6–9. In this example, a programmable CIC version of the same multichannel WDRC hearing aid (Sound FX™) as in Figures 6–7 and 6–8, was fit on a person with a precipitous (noise-induced) hearing loss. The initial fitting was performed according to the NAL-R fitting method (bottom left panel). The hearing aid was measured again when programmed with the same trimmer settings, to determine how NAL-R results would compare to the expectations of the DSL targets (bottom right panel). Both real ear measures were taken on the Audioscan™ real ear measurement system. The settings for NAL-R are close to DSL targets for the low and mid frequencies, but fell short of DSL targets for the high frequencies.

It is difficult to say whether this is a clear indication of the differences between NAL-R and DSL, because a comparison between these two fitting methods is like comparing "apples to oranges" (see Chapter 2). Although NAL-R is concerned with insertion gain, DSL is concerned with in situ output. Furthermore, on the Audioscan™, the input stimuli for these two fitting methods is different; a 55 dB SPL sweep tone was used for NAL-R, to determine that the greatest gain would be present for this relatively low input sound level. For the DSL method, the sweep tone can be presented at 55 dB SPL (to represent soft speech), 70 dB SPL (to represent average speech), and 85 dB SPL to represent loud speech. However, one cannot simply compare NAL-R to DSL using the same stimulus input level, because, according to the Audioscan™ user's guide, the sweep tones for the two fitting methods are different in composition compared to that used for the threshold-based fitting methods, such as the NAL-R fitting method. To represent the long-term average speech spectrum as closely as possible, the sweep tone for DSL is specifically weighted at different frequencies. The sweep tone stimulus for the DSL method is also specifically intended to activate the compression of a hearing aid in a similar manner as speech itself would activate the compression. Neither of these is the case for the sweep tone used to determine gain for the NAL-R fitting method.

Figure 6–10 shows the fitting results of the same CIC-type of hearing aid (same circuit as well) for a person with a moderately-severe high-frequency hearing loss. This time, the trimmers were first programmed to reach as closely as possible to the DSL targets for the person's hearing loss. With the trimmers left in the same position, subsequent measures were taken to determine how the gain would compare to the NAL-R target for the same hearing loss. As shown in Figure 6–9, (bottom-left panel), the output comes close to the DSL targets for the low to mid frequencies, but with the sweep tone input, the output falls nearly 40 dB short of the target for 4000 Hz! As shown in the bottom-right panel, the same trimmer settings result in an overshoot of the NAL-R target for the low to mid frequencies, but fall around 8 dB short of the target gain for 4000 Hz.

The same person with the high-frequency hearing loss was tested again—this time to compare an analog, multichannel WDRC hearing aid to a DSP hearing aid (Figure 6–11). A nonprogrammable DynamEQII™ circuit in a BTE style (Unitron's Sound FX™) was compared to the Oticon Digifocus™ BTE to determine how closely each one could approach the DSL high-frequency targets. Figure 6–10 shows that both hearing aids were quite similar in their high-frequency gain; that is, they both provide similar low-frequency and mid-frequency gain, but

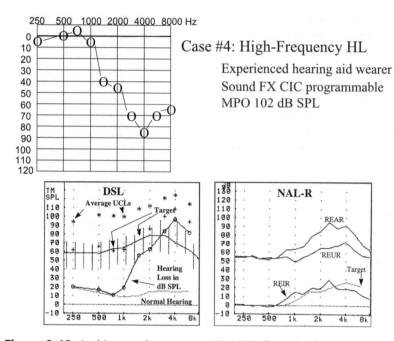

Case #4: High-Frequency HL

Experienced hearing aid wearer

Sound FX CIC programmable

MPO 102 dB SPL

Figure 6–10. In this example, a person with a high-frequency hearing loss was fit with a programmable CIC version of the same multichannel WDRC hearing aid (Sound FX™) as the persons shown in the previous figures. This time, however, the initial fitting was performed according to the DSL fitting method (bottom left panel). Later on, the hearing aid was measured again when programmed with the same trimmer settings, to determine how the DSL results would compare to the expectations of the NAL-R target (bottom right panel). Both real ear measures were taken on the Ausioscan™ real ear measurement system. Note that gain is measured for the NAL-R, while output is measured for the DSL. This stimulus for the NAL-R method was a sweep tone at 55 dB SPL. Again, the stimuli for the NAL-R and the DSL fitting methods are described in the legend for Figure 6–9. With the trimmers set to reach the DSL target, the aided gain exceeds the NAL-R target.

both hearing aids fall 30 to 40 dB short of the high-frequency DSL targets. Although this says nothing about the sound quality comparison between these two hearing aids, it does show that with the DSL 70 dB SPL sweep tone input, a "high-end" analog and a DSP hearing aid both performed similarly for output. The high-frequency gain control for the Sound FX™ was turned up to maximum setting; it is unknown whether the high-frequency gain of the DigiFocus™ could have been turned up higher. It is possible that both hearing aids could have approached the DSL targets if a 3 mm Libby™ horn was used instead of the conventional 13 mm tubing for the earmold.

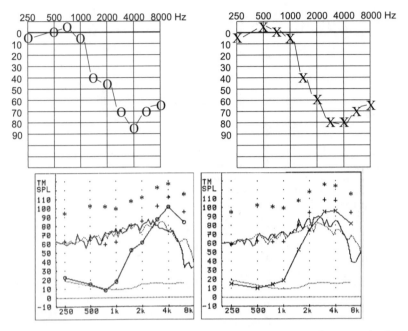

Figure 6–11. Right and left ear fittings according to the DSL fitting method are shown above. Two different hearing aids were tried for a person with high-frequency hearing loss (the same person as in Figure 6–10). The analog Sound FX™ BTE model was compared to a digital BTE of similar power and gain. Both of these hearing aids provide similar output, according to the DSL fitting method, as seen in the bottom panels. Note that both hearing aids fall short of meeting DSL targets, even when set to maximum settings that were comfortable to the client (the Sound FX™ high-frequency gain trimmers were set to their maximum gain. Although this does not deal with the sound quality differences between these two hearing aids, the similarity of their outputs highlights the chasm between the ideals of academia and the realities of hearing aid manufacturing.

A CLINICAL "SPECTRUM" OF HEARING AIDS

Linear peak clipping, output limiting compression, and WDRC can be placed next to each other on a clinical spectrum (see Figure 6–12). Linear peak clipping hearing aids are more similar or closer to output limiting compression hearing aids than they are to WDRC hearing aids. Thus, output limiting is like a bridge between linear peak clipping and WDRC.

A Clinical Spectrum of Amplification

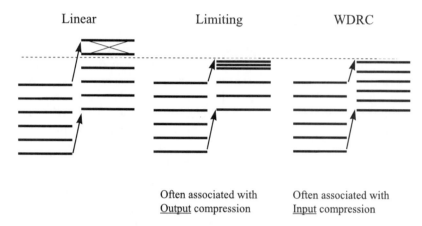

Linear   Limiting   WDRC

Often associated with   Often associated with
Output compression   Input compression

Figure 6–12. For each of three types of hearing aids, two sets of horizontal lines and arrows are shown, with the left lines representing the input, the arrows representing the gain, and the right lines representing the output. The dotted line represents the loudness tolerance level for some particular client. For linear hearing aids, the gain is the same for all input levels. When the output reaches the "ceiling" of loudness tolerance, the output is clipped, resulting in distortion of sound quality. For output limiting hearing aids, only the top "output" lines are squeezed together, because the gain is linear for soft and average input sounds and dramatically reduced for high-intensity input sounds. For wide dynamic range compression hearing aids, both the input and output lines are evenly spread apart because the gain is gradually reduced as the input intensity increases. A large dynamic range is "evenly" shrunk into a smaller one, which restores normal loudness growth. (Figure courtesy of Huup Van den Heuvel, personal communication).

Linear Hearing Aids

Linear hearing aids have enjoyed a wide but diminishing range of fitting applicability; they can provide a lot of gain for severe-to-profound hearing losses or less gain for mild-to-moderate hearing losses. Their most salient feature is that they give the same gain for all input levels. Note on the left-most graphic of Figure 6–12, that soft, average, and loud inputs are all "elevated" by the same amount. The worst thing about this linear type of gain is that the MPO is limited with peak clipping. Sound that is limited in this manner is often distorted and has poor quality for the listener.

Output Limiting Hearing Aids

The output limiting compression hearing aid (usually found together with output compression in general) also can be applied to a wide clinical fitting range. It is often associated with high-power circuitry, however, which provides a lot of gain for the client with severe-to-profound hearing loss. The middle graphic on Figure 6–12 shows that with its high kneepoint of compression and high compression ratio, the output limiting compression hearing aid "elevates" soft and average input levels by the same amount; in this way it is like the linear hearing aid on the left. Unlike the linear hearing aid, however, the output limiting compression hearing aid has a conventional compression control that enables compression to limit the output. This is accomplished without the degree of distortion often associated with linear peak clipping.

WDRC Hearing Aids

The WDRC hearing aid (which is a type of input compression) can also be fit on many different hearing losses, but it often provides less gain than the output limiting hearing aid. The right-most graph on Figure 6–12 shows that with a low threshold kneepoint and low compression ratio, the WDRC hearing aid gives progressively less and less gain as the inputs increase. Recall from Chapter 4 that the focus of WDRC is to restore normal loudness growth by shrinking a large dynamic range into a smaller one. The gain, however, does *not* decrease to the same degree as the input SPLs increase; otherwise the output would remain the *same* for all input levels. The gain must go down more slowly than the input SPLs go up.

When attempting to fit WDRC hearing aids on clients who are accustomed to wearing linear hearing aids, they may initially find that the WDRC hearing aids are "not loud enough." For soft input sounds, the WDRC hearing aids may be satisfactory to these clients because it is for these sounds that they provide the most gain; however, with their low compression kneepoint and low ratio of compression, the WDRC circuit will not provide as much gain as the older linear hearing aids did for average-to-intense input sounds.

Clients who are accustomed to linear peak clipping may therefore, initially reject WDRC. For some, it may be a good idea to fit them with output limiting compression, because this type of compression is closer to linear peak clipping. For new clients with mild-to-moderate SNHL who have never worn hearing aids before, WDRC may provide a very good fit.

At the risk of repetition, it is worth repeating a point made in Chapter 4: output limiting "does its work" above its threshold kneepoint to limit the output, while WDRC "does its work" below its kneepoint to increase the gain for soft sounds.

FITTING HEARING AIDS: THE ART AND THE SCIENCE

The plethora of hearing aid fitting formulas attests to the vastly different issue of fitting the ear versus the eye. Precious little data attest to the correctness of any one hearing aid fitting method as opposed to another. Instead, clinicians are faced with the situation of learning new fitting methods as they appear or become "in vogue."

The late 1980s and early 1990s saw an explosion of new fitting methods, such as Fig6, IHAFF, and DSL. New technology, such as WDRC also became commonplace. Recent knowledge about the workings of the cochlea, as discussed in Chapter 1, have confirmed what many clinicians have long suspected: for SNHL, soft sounds need to be amplified by a lot and loud sounds need to be amplified by little or nothing at all. Restoring normal loudness growth, although not a new concept, has become a rediscovered goal in hearing aid fitting methods, because the compression technology required to do so has now become a reality.

Restoring normal loudness growth with hearing aids means the whole range of SPLs that encompass perceptions of "soft" to "loud" for the normal hearing person must be squeezed into the smaller dynamic range for the person with hearing loss. According to Cox (1995), sounds that are perceived as "soft" by the person with normal hearing need only to be given sufficient gain to make them be perceived as "soft" by persons having hearing loss; "comfortable" sounds for the person with normal hearing need to be given sufficient gain to make them "comfortable" to the person with a hearing loss; and "loud" sounds for the person with normal hearing need to be given sufficient gain to make them "loud" to the person with a hearing loss. This type of amplification is the basic focus of the new suprathreshold fitting methods.

Making the Transition to Suprathreshold Fitting Methods

For those who routinely use threshold-based fitting methods, supra-threshold methods call for a marked departure in clinical orientation/ philosophy. Many clinicians (the author included) who were not originally trained or exposed to suprathreshold-based fitting methods, have difficulty employing them during clinical fittings.

The fundamental concepts of suprathreshold fitting methods are very different from those of threshold-based methods. As was discussed earlier and as Figures 6–9 and 6–10 show, direct comparison between these two types of fitting methods can be very difficult. On the other hand, when entering a hearing loss on real ear test equipment, a direct comparison of required gain for different threshold-based fitting methods (e.g., from POGO, to NAL-R, to Berger, to Libby, etc.) can be quite simple; each one of these methods offers a single target that is based on some mathematical calculation or division of the audiometric thresholds. For any particular hearing loss, one can toggle between these different threshold-based methods quite easily on most real ear test equipment, and the targets for each method can be readily visualized.

A comparison between NAL-R and Fig6 (a suprathreshold fitting method) is also fairly straightforward, because Fig6 is plotted on the same type of gain/frequency graph. Fig6 simply has three targets for three different input levels instead of one target for any one input level.

A comparison between NAL-R and IHAFF or between NAL-R and DSL, however, is not always such a straightforward process (see Figures 6–9 and 6–10). Consider the comparison obstacles that will confront the clinician who wants to compare the gain requirements of DSL with NAL-R. As discussed in Chapter 3, for DSL, the hearing loss and all other values are placed on an "SPL-o-gram" because hearing aids are measured in SPL. Several targets appear on the screen for different input levels as well as for uncomfortable levels. The range of the basic, unaided LTASS may also appear to clutter things further.

DSL also looks at *in situ output*; not insertion gain. DSL is not concerned with aided versus unaided SPL at the eardrum; real ear unaided responses are measured only to obtain real ear-to-2cc coupler differences and these are used in conjunction with the gain of the hearing aid to determine in situ output. Results of amplification are read in terms of *output* rather than gain, because for DSL, the output is what the person is getting as an end product of amplification. If gain is to be determined from DSL, it must be found by subtracting input levels from output levels.

DSL also asks for specific transforms to arrive at a more accurate estimation of actual output in the client's ear. If circumaural headphones are used during testing, DSL requires that the *real ear-to-dial difference* also be calculated for each audiometric test frequency. Insert headphones, on the other hand, are calibrated in a 2cc coupler and so are hearing aids: therefore, this kind of conversion does not apply to insert headphones. Microphone location effects are taken into account for the various different styles of hearing aids (BTE, ITE, CIC, etc). On some real ear test equipment (e.g., Audioscan™), the stimulus during real ear measurement is also unique to DSL.

There is a huge chasm between the ideals to which the new suprathreshold fitting methods aspire and the present "state-of-the-art" technology in hearing aids. Clinicians are often dismayed by a complete inability to reach the aided targets for some suprathreshold fitting methods. Advocates of IHAFF point out that this is common, but that the main idea is to approximate the targets as closely as possible (Van Vliet, 1997). The gulf between targets and actual hearing aid responses can also be encountered when using DSL, especially for pronounced high-frequency hearing losses.

A question that might come to mind is whether the targets, if reached, would be appreciated or accepted by the client wearing the hearing aid in the first place. Can a client always tolerate levels that would theoretically maximize their speech intelligibility? Can a fewer number of hair cells handle the acoustic load required by some of the new suprathreshold-based fitting methods? The difference between the ideals of some suprathreshold fitting methods and the realities that present hearing aid technology can deliver, can become quite evident to the clinician.

Some Philosophy

The philosophy of fitting hearing aids is really found in the fitting methods. The compromise between early linear state-of-the-art technology and small dynamic ranges that gave rise to threshold-based fitting methods was discussed in Chapter 2. The loudness growth philosophy behind many of today's suprathreshold fitting methods was discussed in Chapter 3. Fitting methods, however philosophical they may be, are still a *tool* for conceptualizing a problem and solution. The technology discussed in Chapter 4 is just a means to this end.

Fitting methods should not be put ahead of a client's needs, nor should they be held up as banners of one's stance in a holy war against peers who may use different methods. As discussed in Chapter 2, the whole field of clinical hearing aid fitting is not as purely scientific as we sometimes want to think it is.

Fitting methods are a way to predict what will happen for a client with their hearing aids. But like predicting the weather, there are *many* variables to consider when predicting what hearing aids will do. For clinicians, one issue to consider that has already been discussed, involves the ideals of fitting methods versus the realities offered by the hearing aid technology we have today. A second issue for clinicians, also discussed here, involves the troubles changing from older methods that have underlying assumptions of linear amplifiers to newer ones that assume compression. A third issue for clinicians to consider is choosing which method is the best one. One issue that should never be ignored is excessive output, because, obviously, this can cause further hearing loss.

In general, it may be helpful for clinicians to consider fitting methods as *tools*. In keeping with this imagery, some tools are large and small wrenches, some are screwdrivers, and then there are pliers. It may be a good idea to consider the targets of suprathreshold fitting methods, like DSL, as a goal to eventually and ideally achieve. A new elderly client may not initially accept the amount of gain or output suggested by DSL, however, and in such a case, it may be a good idea to start off by fitting this client with a method that asks for less gain (e.g., NAL-R). The fitting method used should depend on what the goals are. Perhaps clinicians should not slavishly adhere to any one particular fitting method for all cases.

When the client is a child, for example, the fitting method assumes a more decisive and serious role. If the child is prelinguistic, he or she is not able to voluntarily suggested specific alternatives. In addition, audiometric information may be incomplete. The acquisition of language is a fundamental concern for a child who has no language base. The DSL fitting method may be very applicable here because it can prescribe output levels with minimal voluntary information from the client and its focus is the audibility of as many speech sounds as possible.

In many adult cases with mild-to-moderate hearing loss, however, it may not be possible to predict truly what will be needed and finally accepted from a hearing aid fitting. As any "seasoned" clinician knows, there is a lot of room for change in any fitting. Fitting methods, whether suprathreshold-based or threshold-based, are only a means to an end. Is this end optimal speech intelligibility or is it comfort on the part of the listener or both?

From a physiological perspective, it is not presently possible to model what is really going on in the aided cochlea with any one particular fitting method. Most clinicians fit hearing aids to the best of their abilities, but amplification at specific frequencies does not grow new hair cells. Perhaps hearing aids are not a sufficiently sophisticated tool whereby to imitate the exquisite function of the cochlea. Aside from the even more coarse technology offered by cochlear implants, however, hearing aids are all that is available. Aided sound outputs are driven through a middle ear system with the intention of increasing the traveling wave amplitude and stimulating damaged hair cells. The technology of WDRC is meant to imitate the role of the outer hair cells, which are thought to help the inner hair cells sense soft sounds. Hearing aids, however, cannot presently *sharpen* the traveling wave, as the outer hair cells are thought to do. Although our hearts might be in the right place, we are still "picking up needles with mittens on."

Now we come full circle to the initial "big-picture" discussion of what we think we are actually doing when we fit hearing aids. As clinicians, we must be careful not to damage residual hearing with overamplification. For Mrs. McGillicudy who has presbycusis, however, what is the upshot of fitting a hearing aid with one method versus another? What really constitutes a good hearing aid fitting? Are we really doing what we say we are doing when we fit hearing aids with one method versus another? Unlike optometry, various hearing aid fitting strategies abound in our field, but the benefits of each fitting method are not clearly defined. People do not develop a splitting headache or stand a greater chance of driving a car into a tree when fit with NAL-R versus DSL. Hearing aids and people still mix like oil and water. Issues like sound quality and speech intelligibility come into the picture, but it is the clinician's skill at both the art and science of fitting hearing aids that still remains at the heart of the matter.

SUMMARY

■ Hearing aids, even the most sophisticated compression hearing aids, are a coarse, gross approximation of an exquisitely fine-tuned cochlea. This is why the term hearing "aid" is not such a bad one. A hearing aid for an ear is like a cane for a bad knee; it helps, but it cannot replace the real thing. We can no more restore normal cochlear function with a hearing aid than we can replace an amputated hand with an artificial one.

■ Two basic "camps" of hearing aids were outlined: output compression with output limiting compression for severe-to-profound hearing loss and input compression with WDRC for mild-to-moderate SNHL. Within the category of input compression with WDRC, the elements of BILL and TILL were also described. These types of WDRC are important to discuss because people with mild-to-moderate SNHL form the largest portion of our clinical fitting population.

■ Multichannel WDRC circuits that incorporate BILL and TILL in one hearing aid are becoming very popular for use with this large segment of the fitting population. The fitting rationale and controls of a multichannel WDRC hearing aid (the DynamEQ™ by Gennum), was discussed.

■ The art and the science of clinical hearing aid fittings were discussed. In particular, it can be very difficult for clinicians to make the transition from threshold-based to suprathreshold-based fitting methods, and to decide which fitting method to use. Furthermore, there is a large chasm between the ideals of some hearing aid fitting methods and the deliverable realities of most hearing aid circuits. With these situations, the clinical fitting of hearing aids remains both an art and a science.

RECOMMENDED READING

Killion, M. C. (1996, August). Compression distinctions. *Hearing Review, 3*(8), 29–32.

Venema, T. H. (1995). A flexible alternative for difficult hearing loss configurations. *The Hearing Journal, 48*(11), 35–36.

Venema, T. H., (1995, December). Fitting severe to profound hearing loss. *Hearing Instruments, 46*(12), 23–24.

REFERENCES

Armstrong, S. (1996, September). *Chips and dips—an engineering perspective of hearing aid circuits, power supplies, and the like,* Paper presented at Jackson Hole Rendezvous, Jackson Hole, WY.

Anthony, S. 91977, March). *Compression viewed through multi-media glasses.* Paper presented at Seminars in Audition, Ontario, Canada.

Armstrong, S. (1993). The dynamics of compression: Some key elements explored. *The Hearing Journal, 46*(11), 43–47.

Bentler, R. A., & Duve, M. (1997, April). *Progression of hearing aid benefit over the 20th century.* Poster session presented at American Academy of Audiology, Fort Lauderdale, FL.

Berger, K. W., Hagberg, E. N., & Rane, R. L. (1979). Determining hearing aid gain. *Hearing Instruments, 30*(4), 26–44.

Berlin, C. I. (1994). When outer hair cells fail, use correct circuitry to simulate their function. *The Hearing Journal, 47*(4), 43.

Bess, F. H., & Humes, L. E. (1995). *Audiology: The fundamentals* (2nd ed.). Baltimore: Williams and Wilkins.

Bobbin, R. P. (1996). Chemical receptors on outer hair cells and their molecular mechanisms. In C. I. Berlin (Ed.), *Hair cells and hearing aids* (pp. 29–56). San Diego: Singular Publishing Group, Inc.

Borg, E., Canlon, B., & Engstrom, B. (1995). Noise induced hearing loss: Literature review and experiments in rabbits. *Scandinavian Audiology, 24*(Suppl. 40), 117–125.

Brownell, W. E. (1996). Outer hair cell electromotility and otoacoustic emissions. In C. I. Berlin (Ed.), *Hair cells and hearing aids* (pp. 3–28). San Diego: Singular Publishing Group, Inc.

Byrne, D., & Dillon, H. (1986). The national acoustics laboratories' (NAL) new procedure for selecting gain and frequency response of a hearing aid. *Ear and Hearing, 7*(4), 257–265.

Byrne, D., Parkinson, A., & Newall, P. (1990). Hearing aid gain and frequency response requirements for the severely/profoundly hearing impaired. *Ear and Hearing, 11,* 40–49.

Byrne, D., & Tonnison, W. (1976). Selecting the gain in hearing aids for persons with sensorineural hearing impairments. *Scandinavian Audiology, 5,* 51–59.

Carhart, R. (1946). Tests for selection of hearing aids. *Laryngoscope, 56,* 780–794.

Cornelisse, L. E., Gagne, J. P., & Seewald, R. C. (1991). Ear-level recordings of the long-term average spectrum of speech. *Ear and Hearing, 12,* 47–54.

Cornelisse, L. E., Seewald, R. C., & Jamieson, D. G. (1994). Wide-dynamic-range compression hearing aids: The DSL[i/o] approach. *The Hearing Journal, 47*(10), 23-29.

Cox, R. M. (1995). Using loudness data for hearing aid selection: The IHAFF approach. *The Hearing Journal, 48*(2), 10–44.

Cox R. M., & Alexander, G. C. (1995). The abbreviated profile of hearing aid benefit. *Ear and Hearing, 16*(2), 176–183.

Cox, R. M., Alexander, G. C., Taylor, I. M., & Gray, G. A. (1997). The contour test of loudness perception. *Ear and Hearing, 18*(5), 388–400.

Cox, R. M., & Moore, J. N. (1988). Composite speech spectrum for hearing aid gain prescriptions. *Journal of Speech and Hearing Research, 31,* 102–107.

Dillon, H. (1988). Compression in hearing aids. In R. E. Sandlin, (Ed.), *Handbook of hearing aid amplification* (Vol. I). Boston: College Hill Press.

Dillon, H., Katsch, R., Byrne, D., Ching, T., Keidser, G., & Brewer, S. (1998). The NAL-NL1 prescription procedure for non-linear hearing aids. *National Acoustics Laboratories Research and Development, Annual Report 1997/98* (pp. 4–7). Sydney: Australian Hearing, a Commonwealth Statutory Authority, incorporating the National Acoustics Laboratories.

Durrant, J. D., & Lovrinic, J. H. (1984). *Bases of hearing science* (2nd ed.). Baltimore: Williams and Wilkins.

Edmonds, J., Staab, W. J., Preves, D., & Yanz, J. (1998). "Open" digital hearing aids: A reality today. *The Hearing Journal, 50*(10), 54–60.

Engstrom, H., & Engstrom, B. (1988, June). *The ear.* Uppsala Sweden: Widex.

Etymotic Research. (1996). *Fig6 Hearing aid fitting protocol. Operating manual.* Elk Grove Village, IL: Author.

ER-44 D-MIC data sheet. (1997). Etymotic Research, 61 Martin Lane, Elk Grove Village, IL 60007.

Gitles, T. C., & Tillman-Niquette, P. (1995). Fig6 in ten. *The Hearing Review, 2*(10), 28–30.

Gold, T. (1948). The physical basis of the action of the cochlea. *Proceedings of the Royal Society of London, Biological Science, 135,* 492–498.

Hickson, L. M. H. (1994). Compression amplification in hearing aids. *American Journal of Audiology, 3*(3), 51–65.

Hodgson, W. R. (1986). Hearing aid development and the role of audiology. In W. R. Hodgson (Ed.), *Hearing aid assessment and use in audiologic habilitation* (pp. 1–12). Baltimore: Williams and Wilkins.

Hull, R. H. (1995). *Hearing in aging.* San Diego: Singular Publishing Group, Inc.

Independent Hearing Aid Fitting Forum. (1994, August). *A comprehensive hearing aid fitting protocol. User's manual.* [Phone: 714-579-0717].

Jerger, J., Chmiel, R., Stach, B., & Spretnjak. (1993). Gender affects audiometric shape in presbycusis. *Journal of the American Academy of Audiology, 4,* 42–49.

Johnson, W. A. (1993). Beyond AGC-O and AGC-I: Thoughts on a new default standard amplifier. *The Hearing Journal, 46*(11), 37–42.

Kemp, D. T. (1978). Stimulated acoustic emissions from within the human auditory system. *Journal of the Acoustical Society of America, 64,* 1386–1391.

Killion, M. C. (1996a). Compression; Distinctions. *The Hearing Review 3*(8), 29–32.

Killion, M. C. (1996b). Talking hair cells: What they have to say about hearing aids. In C. I. Berlin (Ed.), *Hair cells and hearing aids* (pp. 125–172). San Diego: Singular Publishing Group, Inc.

Killion, M. C. (1997a). A critique on four popular statements about compression. *The Hearing Review, 4*(2), 36–56.

Killion, M. C., (1997b). "I can hear what people say, but I can't understand them." *The Hearing Review, 4*(12), 8–14.

Killion, M. C. (1997c). The SIN report: Circuits haven't solved the hearing-in-noise problem. *The Hearing Journal, 50*(10), 28–34.

Killion, M. C., & Fikret-Pasa, S. (1993). The 3 types of sensorineural hearing loss: Loudness and intelligibility considerations. *The Hearing Journal, 46*(11), 1–4.

Killion, M. C., Schulein, R., Christensen, L., Fabry, D., Revit, L., Niquette, P., & Chung, K. (1998). Real-world performance of an ITE directional microphone. *The Hearing Journal, 51*(4), 24–38.

Killion, M. C., Staab, W., & Preves, D. (1990). Classifying automatic signal processors. *Hearing Instruments, 41*(8), 24–26.

Kuk, F. K., (1996). Real-world consumer satisfaction with a user-controlled, multi-microphone communication system. *Hearing Instruments, 47*(1), 24–28.

Kuk, F. K. (1998). Open or closed? Let's weigh the evidence. *The Hearing Journal, 50*(10), 54–60.

Libby, E. R. (1986). The 1/3-2/3 insertion gain hearing aid selection guide. *Hearing Instruments, 37*(3), 27–28.

Libby, E. R. (1988). Hearing aid selection strategies and probe tube measures. *Hearing Instruments, 39*(7), 10–15.

Libby, E. R., & Sweetow, R. (1987). Fitting the environment-Some evolutionary approaches. *Hearing Instruments, 38*(8), 11–16.

Longwell, T. F., & Gawinski, M. J., (1992). Fitting strategies for the 90s: Class D amplification. *The Hearing Journal, 45*(9), 2–5.

Ludvigsen, C. (1997, March). Basic rationale of a DSP hearing instrument. *The Hearing Review, 4*(3) 58–70.

Lybarger, S. F. (1944). U. S. Patent Application SN 543, 278.

Lybarger, S. F. (1963). *Simplified fitting system for hearing aids.* Canonsburg, PA: Radio Ear Corp.

McCandless, G. A., & Lyregaard, P. E. (1983). Prescription of gain and output (POGO) for hearing aids. *Hearing Instruments, 34*(1), 16–21.

Mueller, H. G. (1997). Prescriptive fitting methods: The next generation. *The Hearing Journal, 50*(1), 10–19.

Mueller, H. G., & Killion, M. C. (1990). An easy method for calculating the articulation index. *The Hearing Journal, 43*(9), 14-17.

Mueller, H. G., & Killion, M. C. (1996). Http://www.compression.edu., *The Hearing Journal, 49*(1), 10–46.

NAL non-linear (NAL NL1) User Manual, version 1.01, National Acoustics Laboratories, 126 Chatswood NSW 2067 Australia, 1998.

Norris, C. H. (1996). Cochlear outer hair cells vis-a-vis semicircular canal type II hair cells. In C. I. Berlin (Ed.), *Hair cells and hearing aids* (pp. 3–28). San Diego: Singular Publishing Group, Inc.

Pavlovic, C., Bisgaard, N., & Melanson, J. (1998). The next step: "Open" digital hearing aids. *The Hearing Journal, 50*(5), 65–66.

Preves, D. (1997, July). Directional microphone use in ITE hearing instruments. *The Hearing Review, 4*(7), 21–27.

Roberts, M., & Schulein, R., Etymotic Research. *Objective measurement of the intelligibility performance of hearing aids.* Based on paper presented at the 103rd Convention at the Audio Engineering Society in New York City, September 26–29, 1997.

Ryals, B. M. (1995). Hair cell regeneration: Is it just for the birds? *The Hearing Journal, 48*(7), 10–83.

Schum, D. J. (1998). Open digital platforms: Opportunities and responsibilities. *The Hearing Journal, 51*(1), 44–46.

Seewald, R. C. (1997). Amplification: A child-centered approach. *The Hearing Journal, 50*(3), 61.

Seewald, R. C. (1995, July). *Hearing aid selection and fitting in children.* Workshop presented by The University of Western Ontario, Department of Communicative Disorders and the Hearing Health Care Research Unit.

Staab, W. J., (December, 1996). Limiting systems in hearing aids. *AAS Bulletin, 21*(3), 23–31.

Stone, M. A., & Moore, B. C. J. (1992). Spectral feature enhancement for people with sensorineural hearing impairment: Effects on speech intelligibility and quality. *Journal of Rehabilitation Research and Development, 29*(2), 39–56.

Thornton, A., & Abbas, P. (1980). Low-frequency hearing loss: Perception of filtered speech, psychophysical tuning curves, and masking. *Journal of the Acoustical Society of America, 67*, 623–643.

Van Vliet, D. (1997, May). *IHAFF protocol.* Paper presented at Canadian Association of Speech-Language Pathologists and Audiologists, Toronto, Ontario, Canada.

Von Békésy, G. (1960). *Experiments in hearing.* New York: McGraw-Hill.

Willott, J. F. (1991). *Aging and the auditory system: Anatomy, physiology, and psychophysics.* San Diego: Singular Publishing Group, Inc.

Yost, W. A. (1994). *Fundamentals of hearing: An introduction* (3rd ed.). San Diego: Academic Press, Inc.

APPENDIX A

Classes of Hearing Aid Amplifiers, A, B, D, and H: Where's Class C?

The most basic way to categorize analog (nondigital) hearing aid amplifiers is to break them down into the *way* in which they amplify or provide gain. The amplifier class is the fundamental block on which the rest of the hearing aid characteristics are built. That a hearing aid provides linear gain or compression is independent of the amplifier class. At the root of any linear or compression hearing aid circuit is the class to which its amplifier belongs.

Each type, or class, of hearing aid amplifier can be either linear or compression. For example, spec sheets from many hearing aid manufacturers show hearing aids available in class A linear, class A compression, class D linear, class D compression, class D WDRC, and so on. WDRC is usually associated with class D, and the K Amp™, as a WDRC circuit, is also built on a class D amplifier/receiver.

Class A amplifiers are the oldest amplifier type. They are also the least expensive. As long as the gain requirements are moderate, the class A amplifier produces low distortion (Longwell, and Gawinski, 1992). The main problem with class A amplifiers is that they constantly use battery power whether they are amplifying an input sound or not. Class A amplifiers are, thus, not the most efficient hearing aid amplifiers.

The reason Class A amplifiers constantly use up battery power is that a "bias" current is necessary from the battery to keep the diaphragm of the receiver at a middle position. The receiver of the hearing aid is the part that "receives" sound from the parts of the cicuit that precede it and sends the sound out into the ear canal of the listener. The diaphragm of the receiver wobbles back and forth and in so doing it transduces or changes the electrical energy of the circuit back into sound for the listener. The diaphragm has to be kept at a middle position so it can vibrate freely on both sides of the middle position. The power required to do this usurps power from the battery for the whole time the hearing aid is turned on. If the diaphragm is not kept at a middle position as it vibrates, it hits the sides of the receiver wall, resulting in peak clipping and distortion.

Class B amplifiers are like two class A amplifiers stuck together, back to back. As a result, they are often larger than class A amplifiers. Each of the two active parts of a Class B amplifier works on opposite "sides" of the alternating sound signal. Due to the equal and opposite actions of the Class B amplifier, the diaphragm of the receiver rests at a center position. No bias current is necessary. Class B amplifiers can provide more gain and output than a class A, because the full battery voltage of the hearing aid is applied to each sideways swing of the diaphragm's "wobble." The diaphragm can thus move in a larger side-to-side motion. This is why class B amplifiers are often referred to as "push/pull" amplifiers and are associated with high-power hearing aids.

Because a bias current is not needed to keep the diaphragm centered, the class B amplifier is more efficient in battery consumption than the class A amplifier. When there is no sound coming into the hearing aid, the class B amplifier does not use up much power. The battery consumption increases only as the signal going through the amplifier increases.

Class C stands for a class of very efficient amplifiers found in high-frequency radio transmitters. This type of amplifier is not at all appropriate for hearing aid circuits, so it is not used. Class C does not stand for compression.

The class D amplifier is unique in that it is integrated into the receiver of the hearing aid. Actually, the class D amplifier is a small class A amplifier housed along with a "pulse width modulator" inside the receiver of the hearing aid. A high-frequency pulse is mixed along with the incoming sound signal and the result is a modulated pulse. This modulated pulse controls the opening and closing of four switches, which in turn control the current that goes through the receiver. Two of the switches allow the positive part of the current to go through, and two of them allow the negative part of the current to go through.

Class D amplifiers are very efficient, which results in relatively low battery power consumption. Similar to the class B amplifier, no bias current is needed to keep the diaphragm of the receiver in a center position. In fact, some power is actually returned to the battery during class D amplifier operation. The full battery voltage of the class D amplifier is applied to each half of the alternating sideways swing of the diaphragm. This results in increased gain and output, which is also similar to class B amplifiers. Other benefits of class D amplifiers in hearing aids is decreased distortion and extended high-frequency emphasis. These can increase the quality of sound for the listener (Longwell, & Gawinski, 1992).

The class H amplifier is a relative newcomer for hearing aids. It is actually a class A amplifier with some special added circuitry. The added circuitry adjusts the typical bias current of a class A amplifier, according to the intensity of the sound input. As the input sound is increased, the bias current (needed to keep the diaphragm in a middle position) is also increased. The class H amplifier is efficient because, like the class B and D amplifiers, its battery power consumption depends on the sound input level and the current the hearing aid really needs to do its job.

There is no such thing as class K. The K stands for Killion, the inventor of the K Amp™.

RECOMMENDED READING

Cornelisse, L. E., Seewald, R. C., & Jamieson, D. G. (1994). Wide-dynamic-range compression hearing aids: The DSL[i/o] approach. *The Hearing Journal, 47*(10), 23–29.

Cox, R. M. (1995). Using loudness data for hearing aid selection: The IHAFF approach. *The Hearing Journal, 48*(2), 10–44.

Gitles, T. C., & Tillman-Niquette, P. (1995). Fig6 in ten. *The Hearing Review, 2*(10), 28–30.

Killion, M. C. (1997). The SIN report: Circuits haven't solved the hearing-in-noise problem. *The Hearing Journal, 50*(10), 28–34.

Killion, M. C. (1996b). Compression; Distinctions. *The Hearing Review 3*(8), 29–32.

Mueller, G. H. (1997). 20 QUESTIONS: Prescriptive fitting methods. *The Hearing Journal, 50*(10), 10–19.

This last reference provides lots of further sources. It also gives phone numbers, faxes, and internet addresses for ordering fitting methods.

A P P E N D I X   B

Fitting Technology: FIG6 in Ten*

By Toni C. Gitles, M.A., and Patty Tilman Niquette, M.A.

Ten questions and their answers are provided about using average loudness data for pre-fitting wide-dynamic-range compression hearing aids such as those using the K-AMP® circuit:

1. WHAT IS FIG6?

FIG6 is a computer-based approach to fitting non-linear hearing aids that have wide dynamic range compression (WDRC), such as, but not restricted to, those with KAMP® processing. Until recently, hearing aid fitting targets were for use only with linear hearing aids, with a single target curve for a single input level.

2. HOW DOES FIG6 WORK?

When entering the patient's audiometric thresholds, the program automatically calculates the fitting curves for low-level sounds (40 dB SPL), moderate level sounds (65 dB SPL), and high level sounds (95 dB SPL). Thus, FIG6 provides three gain and frequency response targets, one for each of three input levels. FIG6 calculates insertion gain targets (REIG) and 2 cc coupler response targets.

Toni C. Gitles, M.A., is director of education at Etymotic Research, Elk Grove Village, IL. Patty Tillman Niquette, M.A., is an audiologist and hearing care consultant.
*Reprinted with permission from *The Hearing Review,* November/December 1995, Vol. 2, No. 10, pages 28 and 30.

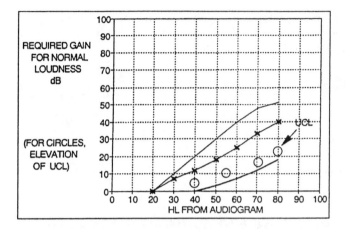

Figure 1. Original "FIG6" diagram. Gain required to restore loudness for low-level (——), comfortable-level (X— X), and high-level (——) sounds. UCL data (O) from Pascoe[6] indicate that the required high-level gain is safe. Reprinted with permission from *The Hearing Journal*, Vol. 46, No. 11 (Killion & Fikret-Pasa[1]).

3. WHY ARE THERE THREE TARGET GAIN CURVES?

The available loudness growth data indicate that individuals with sensorineural hearing loss typically need less gain for intense sounds than for weak sounds. A single target gain curve, therefore, represents a compromise between adequate gain for weak sounds and too much gain for loud sounds. Such a compromise was *required* with linear hearing aids, which lacked the ability to modify their gain and response with level. We now have non-linear hearing aids that change their gain as a function of input level, so a single target makes little sense. More than three would even confuse Mead Killion.

4. WHY WERE 40, 65, AND 95 DB CHOSEN?

An input level of 40 dB SPL represents the weaker elements of conversational speech. FIG6 estimates the gain required to provide aided sound field thresholds of 20 dB HL. (That goal is relaxed for hearing losses above 60 dB HL). A level of 65 dB SPL (50 dB HL) represents conversational speech. A level of 95 dB SPL represents normally loud speech and music. Dennis Van Vliet regularly and effortlessly hits 95 dB and Harvey Dillon's 9-month-old son can produce a 104 dB screech. Hearing aid dispensers converse at 95+ dB levels at national conventions, where the dance bands produce levels of 95–105 dB SPL.

5. WHY IS IT CALLED FIG6?

The name came from Fig. 6 in the article "Three Types of Sensorineural Hearing Loss."[1] The method of calculating gain and frequency response is based on the gain estimates shown in Fig. 6 of that article.

6. WHAT PRINCIPLES DOES FIG6 USE?

It is based on *average* loudness data that relate equal-loudness and threshold curves. Other loudness based approaches, such as the IHAFF approach, use the loudness data of *individual* patients. FIG6 is based on data from several published studies.

7. WHAT ARE THE PUBLISHED STUDIES?

The data of Lippman[2], Lyregaard[3], Hellman and Meiselman[4], and Hellman[5] provide information on how a person with sensorineural hearing loss perceives loudness compared to a person with normal hearing. In addition, Pascoe[6] studied the MCLs and UCLs of 508 ears. Pascoe's MCL data are used to estimate the gain required to restore conversational level speech to the patient's MCL (the 65 dB curve). Mathematical formulas created from these data were used to calculate the level-dependent gain and frequency response appropriate to non-linear hearing aids.

8. SHOULDN'T INDIVIDUAL LOUDNESS CONTOUR TESTS BE PERFORMED?

Ideally, loudness tests should be performed for each hearing aid wearer, but it is not always possible or practical to do so. In most cases, targets based on average loudness growth data provide good first approximations. Individuals with more difficult-to-fit hearing losses, or those for whom amplification has been unsuccessful in the past, may require individual loudness tests.

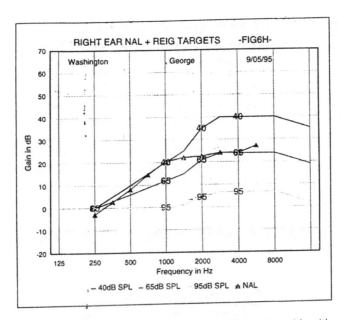

Figure 2. FIG6 target gain curves for WDRC hearing aids with level-dependent frequency response. The target curves (and the NAL-R curve) correspond to the audiogram at the top of Fig.3.

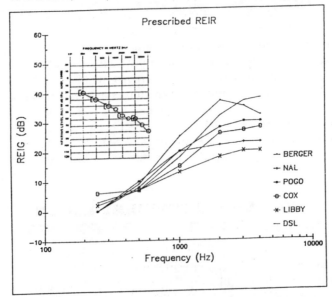

Figure 3. Target gain for fixed-gain, fixed frequency-response hearing aids according to several popular formulae. Reprinted with permission from Singular Publishing Group (Hawkins, Mueller, and Northern[8]).

9. DOES THE DEGREE OF HEARING LOSS MAKE ANY DIFFERENCE?

Yes. Individuals with a hearing loss between 20 and 70 dB HL are normally best served with WDRC hearing instruments. WDRC hearing instrument have also been successful for individuals with more severe hearing loss and reduced intelligibility scores, although an argument can be made that such individuals might be better served with variable recovery time compression *limiting* instruments (see the arguments in "The Three Types of Sensorineural Hearing Loss"[1]).

10. CAN THE DISPENSER UTILIZE FIG6 TO SELECT THE PROPER HEARING AID MATRIX?

Yes. FIG6 calculates 2 cc coupler targets for BTE, ITE, ITC, and CIC hearing instruments. The dispenser uses this information in combination with the manufacturer's published matrices to select the desired hearing aid matrix. *Note:* The appropriate CORFIG curves have been added to the 2 cc coupler curves, so a probe measurement of REIG on a client wearing an ITE, for example, ordered to match the ITE targets should, on the average, match the insertion gain target curves.

More than you may want to know about CORFIG curves is available. The Killion and Revit[7] diffuse field CORFIG corrections themselves can be easily viewed; enter all zeros in the audiogram and select the corresponding 2 cc coupler curve on the pull-down menu.

Acknowledgement
The authors would like to acknowledge the contributions of Don Wilson, Gail Gudmundsen, Mead Killion, and Ed Villchur.

REFERENCES

1. Killion MC and Fikret-Pasa S: The three types of sensorineural hearing loss: Loudness and intelligibility considerations. *Hear J* 1993; 46:11, 31-36
2. Lippman PR, Braida LD and Durlach NI: New results on multiband amplitude compression for the hearing impaired. *J of Acous Soc of America* 1977; 62:S90 {Al.
3. Lyregaard PE: POGO and the theory behind. In Jensen J (ed), *Hearing Aid Fitting: Theoretical and Practical Views*, Proceeds of the 13th Danavox Symposium, Copenhagen 1988:81-94.

4. Hellman RP and Meiselman CH: Rate of loudness growth for pure tones in normal and impaired hearing. *J of Acous Soc of America* 1993;2:966-975.
5. Hellman RP: Personal communication, 1994.
6. Pascoe DL: Clinical measurements of the auditory dynamic range and their relation to formulas for hearing aid gain. In Jensen J, *Hearing Aid Fitting:Theoretical and Practical Views*. Proceedings of the 13th Danavox Symposium, Copenhagen. 1988:129-152.
7. Killion MC and Revit L: CORFIG and GIFROC: Real ear to coupler and back. In Studebaker GA and Hockberg I (eds), *Acoustical Factors Affecting Hearing Aid Performance*, Boston: Allyn & Bacon, 1993: 65-85.
8. Hawkins, DB: Prescriptive approaches to selection of gain and frequency response. In Mueller HG, Hawkins DB and Northern JL (ed): *Probe Microphone Measurements: Hearing Aid Selection and Assessment*, San Diego: Singular Publishing Group. 1992: p 107, Fig. 5-3.

The FIG6 software is available by contacting Toni Gitles at Etymotic Research, 61 Martin Lane, Elk Grove Village, IL 60007; telephone: (708) 228-0006.

A P P E N D I X   C

Compression: Distinctions*

By Mead C. Killion, Ph.D.

Part of the difficulty in fitting compression hearing to instruments is that important distinctions in meaning have been obfuscated by words. Some readers may find the distinctions I use here to be useful:

DISTINCTION #1: COMPRESSION VS. AGC

Humpty Dumpty said to Alice: "When I use a word, it means just what I choose it to mean." "AGC" means different things because writers have sometimes used this generic term to describe specific applications. The words Automatic Gain Control don't specify what *kind* of AGC is meant, so saying "use AGC" is similar to saying "take transportation" without suggesting whether to fly, drive, or call a cab. All bicycles provide transportation. Not all transportation is by bicycle. All wide-dynamic-range compression is AGC, but not vice versa.

DISTINCTION #2: COMPRESSION LIMITING VS. WIDE-DYNAMIC RANGE COMPRESSION (WDRC)

It is often useful to look at *compression limiting* as acting to *reduce* gain above some level, while WDRC acts to *increase* gain below some level.

Mead C. Killion, Ph.D., is president of Etymotic Research, Elk Grove Village, IL, and is adjunct professor of audiology at Northwestern University. He holds degrees in mathematics and audiology.

*Reprinted with permission from *The Hearing Review*, August 1996, Vol. 3, No. 8, Pages 29–30, 32.

That fundamental difference between the two is so important that it is worth saying again in slightly different words Compression limiting acts *above* its threshold to reduce gain for sounds that are too strong, while WDRC acts *below* its (upper) threshold to *increase* gain for sounds that are too weak. It is possible to have both types of compression in one hearing aid: the ReSound hearing instrument, for example, has compression limiting which acts above 50 dB SPL and WDRC which acts below 85 dB SPL.

Compression limiting is used primarily to prevent loud sounds from causing distortion, pain, discomfort, or—in one reported case of a high-powered body aid whose owner's dog barked into the microphone—a ruptured eardrum. Except in the case of the national debt, limiting means "no more beyond a certain amount." In a hearing instrument, "compression limiting" means that the level of sound is not allowed to increase more than a four decibels above the limiting threshold (e.g., a 20 dB further increase in input may be compressed into only a 2 dB increase in output, for example).

Wide Dynamic Range Compression is used to restore audibility for weak sounds and simultaneously restore some of the normal loudness perception that is lost with recruitment. The "wide dynamic range" part comes from the fact that the AGC action is spread out over a 40–50 dB range of inputs, with a gradual change in gain spread out over that range. WDRC has nothing to do with recovery time, as has sometimes been suggested.

Which one is better? Any AGC action can help squeeze the wide range of normal speech levels into the limited range of hearing of someone with hearing impairment, but WDRC comes closer to restoring the normal loudness experience. What is lost with cochlear hearing loss is the increased gain for weak sounds provided by (the mechanical amplification from) normal outer-hair-cell motion. WDRC acts to provide the gain for weak sounds that the impaired ear can no longer provide for itself.

The problem with compression limiting for most types of hearing loss is that it waits too long to do its job: Only when hearing sounds are *almost* too loud does compression limiting come into play. Once limiting is reached, sounds will be *almost* uncomfortable. Limiting does the squeezing job, but with a heavy hand.

Nevertheless, compression limiting appears to be the compression of choice for individuals with 75 dB or greater loss because they often require real-ear output levels within 10–15 dB of their discomfort levels in order to understand speech in noise. Adjusted to limit just below discomfort level compression limiting permits the user to turn the volume control up enough so that all speech sounds fall within the 10 or 15 dB range of outputs required for good intelligibility.[1]

DISTINCTION #3:
TILL VS. MULTICHANNEL COMPRESSION

The typical hearing-impaired individual has a high-frequency loss and needs greater high-frequency emphasis for weak sounds than for strong sounds; in other words he/she needs a TILL or Treble-Increases-at-Low-Levels amplifier. In order to provide this level-dependent frequency response. Villchur[2] and ReSound employed two separate level detection and amplification channels. With the compression characteristics appropriately adjusted for each channel, a TILL response is readily achieved. In the DynamEQ II, a single level-detection circuit controls gain in two amplification channels to achieve the TILL function. In the K-Amp circuit, a single level-detection circuit controls gain in a single amplification channel, but that channel had two electronic functions (treble boost and gain) that can be controlled simultaneously.

In practice, each WDRC circuit can produce a "multichannel" type of level-independent frequency response. Each can be made to produce similar increases in treble boost for weak sounds.

DISTINCTION #4: MULTICHANNEL VS.
MULTICHANNEL VS. MULTICHANNEL

Three distinct "multichannel" operations are possible: Equalization, Detection, and Signal Processing or Compression.

Equalization: Several manufacturers provide multichannel (or band) *equalization,* a frequency-response shaping capability similar to that of the multiband *equalizers* found in some hi-fi amplifiers. The most important practical difference between single-channel and multichannel circuits may be in their frequency-response equalization capabilities; multichannel circuits often allow better tailoring of the response for those with unusual audiometric configurations.

Detection: One difference between single-channel and multichannel detector circuits from an academic standpoint is that a single low-frequency tone can control the entire AGC circuit of a single-detector amplifier such as the K-AMP or DynamEQ II circuits, reducing high-frequency gain as well. The high-frequency gain of amplifiers using 2- or 3-channel detector circuits (e.g., ReSound, 3M), on the other hand, may be relatively unaffected by the narrowband signal.

Despite the theoretical arguments, single-channel detection works quite well in the real world. I have encountered problems resulting from single-frequency tones only rarely (in contrast with their frequent appearance in the laboratory!), presumably because most real-world signals and interfering noises have the same general spectral characteristics as speech. The only user complaints I can recall that have been traced to a single-detector channel have involved the 90–100 dB SPL 25 kHz outputs of ultrasonic motion detectors (The ultrasonic lighting-control system in one well-known multimillion dollar new academic building turns off everyone hearing aids!)

Signal Processing/Compression: Multichannel WDRC compression permits more flexible adjustment of level-dependent frequency-response characteristics because a slope of 18 dB/octave between channels is often possible. Otherwise, a single-channel device works just fine (see Distinction #3 above), and one can even make an academic argument for its superiority: any multichannel compression device risks distorting the normal loudness relationships internal to phonemic speech elements, relationships which provide cues for phoneme identification. A single-channel-TILL compressor provides only a smooth treble boost to the entire phoneme. Although I enjoy the argument, in all fairness, I know of no evidence to support the hypothesis that single-channel compression is inherently superior to multichannel processing.

Mix and Match: The Audio-D (formerly the "Ensoniq" instrument) provides 13 frequency reponse-equalization channels with a single-channel, single-detector K-AMP circuit at the input. The "3-Channel K-AMP" circuit provides fewer equalization channels but much greater slope between channels, again with a single-channel WDRC-TILL K-AMP circuit at the input.

DISTINCTION #5: NONLINEAR DISTORTION VS. NONLINEAR AMPLIFIERS

The term "nonlinear amplifier" causes a lot of confusion because it has been applied to: a) amplifiers that create nonlinear distortion, and b) compression amplifiers that change gain as a function of input level.

Nonlinear (harmonic and intermodulation) distortion is common in poorly designed or overloaded amplifiers, but it does not occur in any well designed AGC system. As Steve Armstrong has pointed out in lectures, any low-distortion AGC must operate as a *linear* amplifier for *waveforms*; an AGC system that "rides gain" so fast as to affect the waveform is effectively clipping!

The nonlinear part of well-designed AGC systems shows up only over time periods. A linear amplifier implies fixed gain as time passes (assuming noone plays with the volume control), while an AGC system *automatically* adjusts the gain over time as a function of input level: slowly enough so as not to distort the sound waveform but fast enough so as not to distort the sound waveform but fast enough to adjust to listening situations.

Even if waveform distortion is avoided, Fikret-Pasa's experiments suggest that it is possible to automatically adust the gain so quickly (using what is called a "short recovery time AGC") that intelligibility in noise is reduced. In her tests with limiting circuits, the industry standard 50 ms recovery time gave poor intelligibility scores, suggesting that we may have focused too much on not recovering quickly *enough*, without realizing that our resultant AGC designs muddy up whole sentences with a recovery that is *too* fast. (The K-AMP design uses a variable-recovery-time circuit that appears to be free of this problem, scoring as well as properly-adjusted linear amplifiers in Fikret-Pasa's experiments.)

Linear aids aren't so bad? Since linear aids still constitute 50% of sales, perhaps the important question is still "why should anyone switch to compression?" The strongest answer is to point out that well-designed compression can relieve the user of the task of constantly adjusting the volume control.

The user with a facile finger can prevent most overload distortion by simply turning down the volume control and make most weak sounds audible by turning it up. I don't think any substantial research has shown any advantage for compression over a properly-adjusted-for-the-circumstances linear amplifier. In hearing instrument research, this has meant a linear hearing instrument with its gain and tone controls set for optimum reception for the text material (usually constant-presentation-level words or sentences)—*but don't stop reading now!*

The problem is that in real life most users don't know how to adjust the gain and tone controls with the skill that research audiologists use during "linear vs. compression" studies. Even users who *can* soon get tired of making constant adjustments. Either way, most users don't bother to "ride gain." *Then* the many disadvantages of linear circuits that are not constantly readjusted (lack of audibility for weak sounds, discomfort and/or distortion for strong sounds) come to the fore. The non-gain-riding user oftens turns down the gain once to avoid discomfort and then can't hear well in quiet or noise. WDRC compression permits the user to attend to other things without any *disadvantage* over an optimally set volume control.

DISTINCTION: #6: COMPRESSION RATIO VS. LOW-LEVEL GAIN INCREASE

I see no point in worrying about compression ratios for fitting hearing aids. Compression ratios *matter*, but they are the hard way of looking at things. Although fitting programs such as FIG6 show compression ratios, they also give targets for low-level gain, speech-level gain, and high-level *gain*. Those *gains* can be most easily set using a multi-curve option on a test box (which will *not* display compression ratios). When those targets are hit correctly, the circuit will have been automatically set to the needed compression ratio. (The compression ratio can be checked, of course, by running an I/O curve and getting out a slide rule.)

When I have a client in front of me, what the client and I are concerned with is nothing more or less than our old friend *gain*. Will there be enough gain for weak sounds to make them audible? Will there be too much gain for strong sounds so they hurt? Will normally loud sounds be loud but not uncomfortable?

Those of us who carry pencils in our pockets and loudness-growth curves (with hearing loss as parameter) in our heads find compression ratios useful because they help us design circuits. We know that a 40 dB cochlear loss typically shows about a 2:1 increase in slope over the normal loudness-growth curve, so that an amplifier with approximately a 2:1 compression ratio will restore the aided loudness-growth curves to normal (and is consistent with Ruggero and Rich's physiological data for loss of outer-hair-cell-amplifier function). A 60 dB loss typically shows a 3:1 slope in loudness growth.[1] In practice, somewhat lower compression ratios than these theoretical values are prescribed by existing fitting targets (and chosen subjectively).

DISTINCTION #7: INPUT VS. OUTPUT COMPRESSION

Don't worry about this one: If you freeze the volume control with tape, you can't tell which is which anyway.

OK, my editors say I should mention that, limiting is used, there is a theoretical advantage for properly-set *output compression* (the control circuit is introduced *after* the volume control), because it gives the user the freedom to choose gain for weak sounds, by adjusting the volume control, without worrying about discomfort.

Most WDRC circuits use input compression, permitting the user to choose the desired gain for strong sounds by adjusting the volume control; weaker sounds are automatically given greater gain by the WDRC action.

One other combination has been popular since the 1970s: compression-limiting circuits with input compression, typically adjusted for action above 65–70 dB SPL (i.e., for a limiting threshold of 65–75 dB SPL at the input, above which the output would increase very little). The term "input compression aid" has traditionally meant such a compression-limiting input-compression circuit.

DISTINCTION #8: WDRC+LINEAR VS. WDRC+LIMITING

One final distinction may be useful. In commercial WDRC hearing instruments, there are three different types of I/O behavior observed once the input SPL rises above approximately 85 dB:

1. Change to linear (K-AMP);
2. Continuation of the same WDRC Compression (e.g., Dyn-Aura, Omni, many more recent 2:1 circuits); and
3. Change to compression limiting (e.g., ReSound).

Where restoration of normal loudness is desired, #1 (high-level linear operations) is indicated, since most impaired loudness-growth curves exhibit complete or partial recruitment (return to normal or near-normal loudness) at about 85 dB SPL. Where protection of someone with moderate-severe hearing loss from discomfort is indicated, #3 (high-level compression limiting) is indicated. Characteristic #2 is a reasonable compromise between the two.

REFERENCES

1. Killion M.C. & Fikret-Pasa S: The three types of sensorineural hearing loss: Loudness and intelligibility considerations. Hear Jour 1993;46(11):31-36.
2. Villchur E: Signal processing to improve speech intelligibility in perceptive deafness. J Acoust Soc Am 1973;53:1646-1657.
3. Fikret-Pasa S: The effects of compression ratio on speech intelligibility and quality. PhD thesis. Northwestern University. Ann Arbor, MI: University Micro films, 1993.
4. Ruggero, M.A. and Rich N.C.: Furosemide alters organ of Corti mechanics: Evidence for feedback of outer hair cells upon the basilar membrane Jour of Neuroscience 1991;11(4):1057-1067.

A HISTORICAL NOTE ON COMPRESSION

WDRC goes back to the 1930's when transatlantic cables were being laid on the ocean floor and talking movies were just starting. Bell Telephone Laboratories' scientists Mathes and Wright[1] (1934) described the use of "companders": *compressors* to increase the signal level of quiet sounds before they began their underwater voyage and *expanders* at the receiving end to restore normal speech levels and loudness variations. Once Steinberg and Gardner[2] (1938) had discovered recruitment and measured the input-output loudness curves of hearing-impaired ears, they commented that the impaired ear acted just as if it had an electronic input expander (like the receiving end of transatlantic telephones), and what was needed to correct for this loss was a compressor in the hearing aid. In their time, "compressor" meant only wide-dynamic-range compressor.

Hy Goldberg in 1965 appears to have been the first to make a high-quality wide-dynamic-range circuit for a BTE hearing aid. Interestingly enough, the problems of proper fitting and counseling with this aid appear to have been one factor in its relatively limited acceptance.

In 1973, Villchur[3] published the results of his own laboratory experiments comparing linear amplification with wide-dymamic-range compression amplification (combined with appropriate post-compression frequency-response tailoring). The dramatic intelligibility improvements he saw, especially in noise, later led Fred Waldhauer of Bell Laboratories and the present author to independently devise high-quality wide-dynamic-range compression amplifiers suitable for hearing aids. The former became the ReSound circuit and the latter became the K-AMP circuit. Other WDRC circuits followed, the most recent probably being the DynamEQ II developed by Steve Armstrong and his colleagues.

REFERENCES

1. Mathes and Wright: Companders. *Bell Syst. Tech. Jour.* 1934;13:315.
2. Steinberg JC and Gardner MB: (1937). The dependence of hearing impairment on sound intensity. *J Acoust Soc Am* 1937;9:11-23.
3. Villchur E: Signal processing to improve speech intelligibility in perceptive deafness. *J Acoust Soc Am* 1973:53:1646-1657.

Index